The Ayurvedic Guide to Polarity Therapy:

Hands-on Healing

A Self-Care Guide

By Amadea Morningstar, MA, RPP

Illustrations by the Author

LOTUS PRESS

DISCLAIMER:
This book is not intended to treat, diagnose or prescribe. The information contained herein is in no way to be considered as substitute for your own good common sense, or as a substitute for a consultation with a duly licensed health care professional.

Library of Congress Cataloging-in-Publication Data
Morningstar, Amadea
The Ayurvedic Guide to Polarity Therapy: Hands-On Healing
ISBN: 0-914955-94-2
I. Subject   I. Title
Library of Congress Control Number: 00-134349

Published by:
Lotus Press
P.O. Box 325
Twin Lakes, Wisconsin 53181
Web: www.lotuspress.com
E-mail: lotuspress@lotuspress.com
(800) 824-6396

Cover, page design and layout: Kerry Jobusch, KPComm

With thanks to CRCS Publications for permission to reprint the following charts: CHART NO.2: CHART OF THE SUBTLE PRANA CURRENTS IN THE HUMAN BODY AND THEIR CHAKRAS AS WHIRLING PRIMARY FUNCTIONAL CENTERS OF ENERGY. CHART NO.1: PYCHO-PHYSIOLOGICAL KEY CHART ANCIENT AND MODERN FOR POLARITY THERAPY. CHART NO.17: THUMBS AS NEUTER RE-FLEXES EMBRACING THE ENTIRE AREAS BELOW THE DIAPHRAGM ON EACH SIDE OF THE BODY, COMPARED TO REFLEXES AROUND THE OUTSIDE OF THE ANKLES AS THE NEGATIVE POLE. CHART NO. 5: THE EMBRYO (FETUS) IN THE MOTHER'S WOMB, WOVEN BY THE ENERGY LINES OF THE FOUR ELEMENTS IN THEIR THREE-FOLD ACTION. and photographs: Dr. Randolph Stone at 60, and in his eighties. Selected quotes throughout the book are also reprinted by arrangement with CRCS Publications, P.O. Box 1460, Sebastopol, CA 95472.

TABLE OF CONTENTS

A DAY WITH HEALING ENERGY

CHAPTER I: WAKING

CHAPTER II: MOVEMENT

CHAPTER III: BREATH

CHAPTER IV: STILLNESS

CHAPTER V: NOURISHMENT: HEALING WITH FOOD

———•———

ACKNOWLEDGEMENTS:

The Ayurvedic Guide to Polarity Therapy: Hands-on Healing

Many people have generously shared their time in support of this book. I want to thank them here.

Dr. Jim Said, DC, ND, RPP, provided core knowledge and clarification about Polarity Therapy that was crucial for the development of this work. Jim Said and Cindy Rawlinson, RPP, LAc, together communicated a vision of Polarity Therapy which deepened mine considerably. Also, their knowledge of the currents, along with the generous sharing of Charmaine Lee, RPP, began to bring these to life for me. Charmaine graciously reviewed the movement chapter in depth, as well. Dr. David Frawley, DOM, was unfailingly kind and supportive in strengthening my understanding of Ayurveda; he has provided an eloquent foreword. Rose Diana Khalsa was equally open in providing her heart-felt foreword from the Polarity Therapy perspective.

Clare Bonser, LMT, RPP, RCST candidate, heretofore simply to be known as "Saint Clare" was the book's last-minute midwife, sparking its arrival on Lotus Press's doorstep when it looked like it could be becalmed in my computer indefinitely. For her generosity and keen editing I am most grateful. Zenia Victor, alias "Saint Zenia" in the sisterhood of the book, provided essential support, proofreading, and visual perspectives. Both Clare and Zenia's keen wits as well as keen eyes are much appreciated. Many people graciously took time to model for the illustrations, including Gordon and Iza Bruen, Ronaldo Estevan, Laurie Forbes, Nick and Amanda Garcia, Louise Henry, Michele Herling, Katherine Mortimer and Bob Bruen. Graphic illustrator Angela

Werneke offered crucial guidance in the development of the final drawings; I thank her deeply. Catherine Weser, graphic artist and computer whiz, provided a similar role in the development of the charts and graphs; her generosity is much appreciated.

David Frawley, Margo Gal, and Ivy Blank gave critical support in Ayurveda for which I am most grateful. Margo's enthusiasm for this integrative look at Ayurveda and Polarity Therapy meant a great deal to me. Melanie and Bob Sachs offered clarity and wisdom in Ayurveda, as well as perspective on Tibetan Buddhist practices, which I much appreciated. Lorin Parrish provided an early assessment of the manuscript which simultaneously supported it and challenged me to reach deeper; I thank her for her honesty and courage. Ron Splude, KinTree Whitecloud, Maureen O'Brien, and Jeremiah Weser gave feedback on chapter 8 at crucial points in its unfolding. Edith Hathaway, Vedic astrologer, generously took time out to look at Dr. Stone's use of metals in healing. Ellie Simmons, RPP, and Gary Peterson, RPP, at APTA kindly helped me make connections with Polarity Therapists at home and abroad; all of whom I'd like to thank for their willingness to share their resources. Nicolai Bachman, Sanskrit and computer educator, helped me into a new computer as my old one was dying. Joe Bisagna and his family at Quik Send copying and packing services saved me more than once, with efficiency and humor.

Suzanne Getz, LMT, RPP, Moksha Kolman, LMT, RPP, Damon Fazio, ND, RPP, LMT, Cynthia Pierro, RMT, RPP, and Rose Diana Khalsa, RPP, offered inspiration both in their practice and teaching of Polarity Therapy, which I much appreciate.

I want to warmly thank Cathy Hoselton at Lotus Press, my publisher Santosh Krinsky, and Kerry Jobusch of KPComm, for their commitment to excellence.

I want to thank all my teachers, family, friends, students, and clients, as well as the difficulties that arose along the way. Thank you for this chance to share. The responsibility for any errors rests with me, of course.

And with much gladness I thank the musicians: Gordy Bruen, Bob Bruen, and Bill Boaz, Iza Bruen, Fats Waller, and Mari Boine. They lit my way with much love.

———•———

FOREWORDS

We live in an age of energy evidenced by the mass media, rapid communication, easy travel and the computer revolution. We no longer see ourselves as fixed beings tied to a particular place or a single job for our entire lives. We see ourselves in relationship, on the move, as dynamic beings possessing a diverse expression in shifting parameters of time and space. This understanding is extending into the field of health as well. We no longer consider ourselves to be mere physical bodies but have a sense of ourselves as an energy field composed of body, mind and spirit.

Based on this recognition, energetic and vibrational forms of healing are becoming more important than simple physical healing modalities. We want to know not just what heals the body on a structural and organic level but what connects us to higher forms of vitality and creativity. We are all seeking the energy not only for bodily health and flexibility but to fulfill our manifold and changing roles in this ever-changing world.

Polarity Therapy is a modern energetic healing practice, with its roots in the yogic teachings of India. It is based upon an understanding of prana, the primary life-force and its manifestation. Polarity Therapy develops the energy side of healing into a profound system of bodywork and subtle energy balancing. It shows us how to master the workings of prana for optimal health and vitality.

Ayurveda is the science of life itself (Ayur is a synonym for "prana" and Veda means "wisdom"), the traditional natural healing system that evolved out of the yogic teachings of India. It contains a comprehensive set of health practices from diet and herbs, to surgery, bodywork, energy work, psychology and meditation. It encompasses all activities of body and mind from a perspective of consciousness. As

Ayurveda and Polarity Therapy systems are related in origin, terminology and inspiration it is only natural to look at both together, which is through the healing energy of prana.

Prana is ultimately the energy of consciousness that flows into manifestation from the Absolute. It is the Divine force of life, love, light, growth and evolution that carries us forward and upward in our manifestation. Underlying our physical body is a field of prana that nourishes, sustains and completes it. Behind the mind is a higher energy field that gives us the power to think and to feel. This energy has its own intelligence. Prana keeps the body functioning when we sleep, supports the immune system and sustains the healing process. Through prana we can facilitate all transformations, including healing that is almost miraculous in its results.

Amadea Morningstar is a prolific and in depth writer on health from an Ayurvedic standpoint. Her two cookbooks—*The Ayurvedic Cookbook and Ayurvedic Cooking for Westerners*—are perhaps the most important books on their subject. *The Ayurvedic Guide to Polarity Therapy*, her new book on Ayurveda and Polarity Therapy is a similarly important work. The Ayurvedic connections with Polarity Therapy, though generally known, are seldom specifically explained. The relevance of Polarity Therapy to Ayurveda, though often noted, is seldom practically taught.

Amadea shows the interface of both systems in great detail. Through her synthesis students of Ayurveda can easily access Polarity Therapy and begin to integrate its many healing methods into their practices. Similarly, students of Polarity Therapy can begin to integrate Ayurveda and its many healing modalities into their practices as well. However, Amadea does not provide a mere naïve equation of the two systems. She notes both their similarities and their differences and respects the unique value of each as a healing discipline in its own right, so that the reader can benefit best from each.

Amadea explains how the teachings of Polarity Therapy relate to the concepts of the elements, gunas, and dhatus that occur in Ayurveda and to Ayurvedic therapies of diet, herbs and exercise. The five elements on which both systems are based are not mere inanimate substances but the basic vibrational rates of all phenomena in the universe, from inanimate matter to the highest reaches of the mind. The elements are imbued with life-energy in our bodily system and serve to transmit the cosmic forces that sustain our existence.

Yet *The Ayurvedic Guide to Polarity Therapy* is no mere comparative study of Ayurveda and Polarity; it is a creative integration and development of both. Her approach is systematic and in-depth, following classical yogic models to project new forms of understanding. She focuses on the three gunas of sattva, rajas and tamas, the universal powers of balance, movement and completion, as the basis for her presentation. The gunas are the prime forces of Mother Nature. Revealing them in the movement of our lives, Amadea adds a new dimension to all the factors of wellness.

The Ayurvedic Guide to Polarity Therapy is a notable compendium, if not encyclopedia of nutrition, herbology, bodywork, psychology, and even astrology, taking the best not only in Ayurveda and Polarity Therapy but in other forms of natural healing as well. It explains these teachings in terms of daily practices and life-style routines that are useful for everyone, with many helpful hints, recipes and formulas that make her work a valuable reference guide for the entire family. It is a wonderful reference book that will be helpful to its readers for many years to come.

The Ayurvedic Guide to Polarity Therapy is a significant book not only for students of Ayurveda and Polarity Therapy but for all those who want to improve their energy on both physical and mental levels. It shines new light on all the main factors of healing from food to emotions. Its readers are bound to come away with many helpful tools to improve the quality as well as duration of their lives.

DR. DAVID FRAWLEY
Author, *Yoga and Ayurveda, Ayurvedic Healing, Ayurveda and the Mind,* etc.

FOREWORD FROM ROSE DIANA KHALSA, R.P.P.

In our society, there is a sickness that is epidemic. It is something you can see in the eyes. It's on CNN and you can read about it in newspapers. It is the sickness of the spirit. So many people in our culture are looking outside of themselves for something that will take away their pain. Something to numb them out, using drugs, food, sex, alcohol. It is very sad.

We need to connect with our spirit, the God within ourselves. The more this grows, the stronger we become. The stronger the light within, the more compassion we can have for others and mostly for ourselves. This is the beginning of healing.

Living in the new millennium, the Aquarian Age, is about bringing vision, community, and deep compassion to the masses. Part of this picture is learning a healthy way of living that will support our spiritual life. Along with this, more and more people are looking for alternative/holistic medicine for answers to their health problems. The truth is, most of the "New Age" techniques are ancient healing modalities, used for centuries to heal.

There was a man named Dr. Randolph Stone, who brought one of these healing modalities to the planet. I believe he was a visionary. One of my Elder teachers told me that when a person's crown chakra is open to the divine, this person has the ability to leave something on the planet that will never be forgotten. Dr. Stone brought an incredible knowledge and understanding of how to see the body and a holistic approach to energy medicine. This modality is called Polarity Therapy.

Polarity Therapy weaves in a beautiful tapestry, ancient wisdom of Ayurveda, Chinese medicine, along with yoga, bodywork, nutrition and self-awareness. One of the things I love the most about Polarity Therapy is its self-help techniques. Taking responsibility for our health is very empowering. This book will gently help with tools for healing yourself.

The Ayurvedic Guide to Polarity Therapy is a book to inspire you, revitalize you, and is a toolbox for jumpstarting your body, mind and spirit. Amadea Morningstar is truly an inspiration! This book will make you laugh and sink into yourself. It is a gentle reminder of the ancient ways of healing.

Amadea will walk you through a beautiful garden of teachings that she has personally practiced. The combination of Ayurveda and Polarity Therapy fits like a glove and is a deepening relationship with food, done with mastery and grace.

Read this book! Take it in. Share the teachings, and most of all, walk your talk, live your truth and come from the heart. Feel your spirit growing with love, respect and spiritual integrity.

Thank you Amadea. May your words touch many. May the wisdom go deep, and help us to remember to laugh, dance, sing, and tell the stories of our healing journey.

Namaste,

ROSE DIANA KHALSA, R.P.P.
Teacher and Practitioner

INTRODUCTION

This book is based on a few assumptions. One is, you don't have to be sick to take care of yourself. Another is, if you are sick, there's a good chance there is something here that will help you ease your difficulties. And you may discover something about Ayurveda and Polarity Therapy, two remarkably effective healing arts.

In my own journey, seven years ago I was asked to teach Ayurvedic nutrition to a group of students studying to become Registered Polarity Practitioners. While well-versed in Ayurveda, I didn't know much about Polarity Therapy, just what I had read in Richard Gordon's fine book, *Your Healing Hands*, as a young massage enthusiast in the 1970's. From him I gathered what some of the magic of Polarity must be. Combining this with my own experiences with energy and healing, it was not hard for me to realize that our hands have energy and can be consciously used for healing. That is as far as my understanding of Polarity Therapy went at that point. At the same time I was fortunate to have as a dream teacher and bodywork practitioner, Shamaan Ochaum. As a young nutrition science grad from Berkeley and Stanford, I was shocked to find that massage was more than massage: that images, electric impulses, and strong rushes of energy enveloped me in something like a healing cocoon. What Shamaan did was her own rare blend of East and West. Under her tutelage, I had to redefine what I thought healing and the body were.

Professionally, I have been associated with food and therapeutic nutrition for many years. And yet in my own life, as in everyone's, nourishment is only part of the picture. In my thirties I discovered that craniosacral therapy and hiking worked well for me in my pregnancy. And in my forties, a back injury which had become painfully chronic gradually healed with the help of Rolfing and Feldenkrais. Touch and movement have been key parts of my healing throughout my life.

As a Western nutritionist, I got fascinated by the East Indian system of Ayurveda in the early 1980's. I was intrigued enough with this vast and potent system to write several healing cookbooks and to integrate its concepts into my teaching and practice. Ayurveda's nature-based approach speaks to me deeply. Yet by the time I began teaching in the Polarity Therapy program at the New Mexico Academy of Healing Arts here in Santa Fe, New Mexico, I was restless to explore new ways to practice. I was no longer content to sit and simply talk about food and herbs with my clients or students.

Several events or processes influenced me. As a nutritionist, I had often worked with people with cancer, as food can be a powerful therapeutic in meeting the disease. Working with cancer on a daily basis, I realized in the early 1980's that I knew very little about death. As this was part of the possibility in many cancers, I wanted to meet it more fully, acknowledge its potential in the equation of healing. Being young and mobile, I hired on as a cook-housekeeper in the Carmel Valley hospice in California. I was a terrible housekeeper and an empathetic confidante. Struggling to keep my balance in the intensity of needs and feelings which the dying process evoked both in the hospice residents and myself, I would come home each night close to devastation. My housemate and friend, artist Dolores Chiappone kept urging me to paint as a way to meet the challenges. I resisted; I knew I was no artist. "It doesn't matter" she kept insisting with her Sicilian clarity, "just do it." Finally I began, and I was shocked to find it was healing. For the next fifteen years, when I was in turmoil or depression, I often painted my way through it.

In the mid-1980's, the hospice had closed and I was back in practice in Santa Fe. I enrolled in a graduate program in transformational counseling at Southwestern College at night. Under the guidance of Drs. Robert Waterman and Marylou Butler, I found myself exploring more about how art, movement, and archetypes can be a part of healing, in a strongly experiential program. As most of us have discovered, it's one thing to know what one needs to do, and quite another to actually be able to hold with oneself to do it. The counseling program encouraged me to help myself more skillfully, as well as to support my nutrition clients to make the changes they wanted.

So by the time I was hired to teach Ayurvedic nutrition to Polarity Therapy students in 1993, I routinely used art and counseling processes as ways to access healing with food. And yet, in the professional Ayurvedic health care community of which I am a part, "practice" is still defined primarily as educational consultations about food and herbs. Other Ayurvedic educators, inspired by the teaching of Dr. Sunil Joshi and Dr. Vasant Lad, have gone on to train in Pancha Karma, the five Ayurvedic actions of cleansing, including therapeutic steams and massage. While I was impressed with their results, this did not seem to be the path for me as a professional. Instead, I have been drawn to learn more about plants and Ayurvedic gardening (another story). Yet there was this nagging sense of limits within my practice. If I didn't want to sit and talk about food any more, how did I want to work?

I learned from my Polarity students that the originator of Polarity Therapy, Dr. Randolph Stone, used bodywork, movement, awareness, and food all as part of his therapeutics. And so did they. Some were working with dance, others were involved with nursing, psychotherapy, and yoga, all loved the bodywork, and they were all exploring. Their learning was an adventure which drew me to consider this exploration, too.

I signed up for ten Polarity sessions at the student clinic with Sister Mary Ann Szydlowski, and began to understand more the whys and wherefores of my early healing experiences with Shamaan. As I trained in the methods myself under the skilled guidance of Moksha Kolman, LMT, RPP and Damon Fazio, ND, RPP, I found rather than being tired after giving a bodywork session, I was energized by the Polarity Therapy, as were my client-partners. Intuitively, it helped me make sense of my life. It was fun. And then I began to integrate it with what I knew about Ayurveda.

Working with healing energy in this broader way lead me to write this book. Many people have barely heard of either healing art, let alone have considered using these simple methods in their own lives. Others will see their similarities with other traditional healing methods they may have learned with their grandmothers or within community. Teaching in Polarity Therapy programs, I found that while many Polarity Therapists respect Ayurveda as an ancient mother to their art, most don't know much about its specific tenets and practices. And most Ayurvedic practitioners have no clue that Polarity Therapy integrates effectively into Ayurveda, and that Polarity techniques can be used to balance the doshas and affect immediate healing. Because Ayurveda has gotten better coverage in recent years, more of the focus in this book is on Polarity Therapy, and how the two sciences can be used for practical healing.

It is in a spirit of adventure that I invite you to join me. In my own life, it's time for a change. One specific example: about ten years ago, therapeutic herbalist Daniel Gagnon and I collaborated on a compact book about colds, flus, bronchitis, and other respiratory challenges. In addition to herbal and nutritional information, we offered specific healing images for each disorder, in the hopes of supporting healing through as many modalities as possible. Many people have told us the book has helped them. And yet I wouldn't do it quite that way anymore, one visualization for each disease. We are each too different. Healing images and symbols do work; they are very powerful. Yet each of us is unique and comes to healing in our own way, with our own dreams and images. There is no one effective system or image for healing; there are many. The challenge lies in discovering the appropriate images and paths for ourselves.

Marc Ian Barasch offers a funny and apt picture of what it can be like to grapple with healing for oneself in a recent interview in *The Sun*. He is talking about illness, and yet for me this could just as easily be applied to habit, addiction, obsession, or other potential facts of life. Here's how he put it:

"I could have communicated with this new partner (his illness), this other to which I was now chained, like in an old movie where two escaped convicts are chained together: you may think you can knock the other guy into a river without getting dragged in yourself, but you can't. In the movies, the outcome is always that the convicts wind up talking to and learning from each other. Having exhausted all other options, they actually discover who the other is. Perhaps I needed to listen to my disease, and to the organ itself..." *"Body Language: A conversation with Marc Ian Barasch on Illness and Healing"* by Derrick Jensen, *The Sun*, January 2000, issue 289.

There's a certain give and take in working with yourself and healing energy, as well as adventure. There's a good amount of information in this book about Ayurveda and Polarity Therapy. And yet what you draw from it will be your own, reflecting your unique relationship to healing.

I wish us the best in all our healing journeys.

In gratitude,

AMADEA MORNINGSTAR,
Santa Fe, NM
February, 2000

HOW TO USE THIS BOOK

Each chapter synopsis is framed in the form of open-ended questions, to invite you to consider your own situation, your relationship to healing energy. The book as a whole is set up as if we were moving through a day together, waking, stretching, breathing. Each chapter addresses issues within the cycle of one day. Information is offered to help make the practices understandable from a larger perspective. This includes sections about the elements, the energy currents, and prana. You can read it all or skip to the boxes, which contain the self-care practices. Or skip the boxes, and simply absorb the philosophical overview. It's up to you.

The RESOURCES list you will find at the end of each chapter is far from inclusive. It is a start toward being able to network with others, or pursuing more learning on your own. I've listed programs or people who have been quoted in the text so you can follow up with them, or texts I know personally and have found helpful. Yet there are literally dozens of fine programs in Polarity Therapy and Ayurveda and hundreds of practitioners that are not mentioned here. To track down more information about programs or practitioners in your area, refer to the listings of national organizations in the RESOURCES section following the next chapter.

ABOUT THESE TWO APPROACHES TO HEALING

ABOUT AYURVEDA:

Ayurvedic medicine is an indigenous healing system of India. It dates back at least four to five thousand years, and is perhaps even older than that. It was originally preserved in the Vedas, the ancient oral tradition of India, and chanted as a way of both remembering and embodying the medicine. Prayer, mantra, breath, and ritual were important parts of the early healing, and were transmitted in Sanskrit. Later, more information was passed on about substances, about plants and animals as well as astrology. Even later, information was added about the healing power of minerals. (1) There are still some families in India who continue to chant one or more of the four Vedas by memory alone, as their way of perpetuating this ancient tradition.

Today Ayurveda works with food, herbal medicines, bodywork, exercise and yoga, cleansing and building techniques, breath, mantra, astrology, and gemology. It can be used either as a self-healing process or by visiting professional practitioners for assessment and education. At the core of its treatment methods lays an ancient understanding of the elements, the mental qualities known as the *gunas*, and the biological energies called *doshas*. We will be exploring all of these in the chapters that follow.

If you are interested in learning more about this tradition, there is a wide range of excellent books listed in the RESOURCES section at the end of this chapter.

ABOUT POLARITY THERAPY:

Polarity Therapy is based on the concept that energy underlies matter, and to effect any lasting changes in health, one must work with the underlying energetic patterns. Energy can be contacted through touch, movement, sound, thought, feelings, and all of the five senses.

This energy underlying health and life has had many names: "prana" in Ayurveda and Yoga, "chi" in traditional Chinese medicine, "manna" in Hebrew mysticism, "bioplasmic energy" or simply "bioenergy" by the Russians of the last century, to name a few (2). Dr. Randolph Stone, the originator of Polarity Therapy, called this energy by its ancient yogic name, "prana".

Having immigrated to the US from his native Austria as a child in 1903, Randolph Stone trained as a "drugless healer" in Chicago in the early part of the twentieth century, becoming a doctor of osteopathy, chiropractry, naturopathy, naprapathy (water therapies), and neuropathy. From an early age he was intensely interested in spiritual and mystical pursuits, as well as medicine. He was an active student of Vivekananda's teachings, Manly P. Hall's Philosophical Research Society, Rosicrucianism, Sufism, the Bible, the Kaballah, and the Koran. In his lifetime, major discoveries came in physics about the atomic structure of life. All of this inevitably influenced his explorations of medicine.

As a physician, Stone tended to probe for the causes underlying the problems he saw in his patients. He asked why some patients returned repeatedly for the same physical adjustment, although it had been done apparently correctly. He was familiar with the chakra system of ancient India, from his spiritual studies and his interest in Ayurvedic medicine. In his work, he began to discover that the energetic system of the chakras gave rise to orbiting energetic currents just off the surface of the physical body, and that he could feel and contact these with his hands. These currents orbited the body much as the newly discovered electrons circled the nucleus of an atom. He was extremely excited to discover this "wireless anatomy" of the body, and over the next sixty years of his practice, he would work to elucidate more specifically what these currents were and how they might be used for healing.

He concluded at one point, *"Energy must flow. Sore spots are blocks in the energy currents. The science and skill come into play in FINDING OUT WHERE THE ENERGY IS BLOCKED AND IN KNOWING HOW TO RELEASE IT. When the current is re-established, the pain leaves at once and normal action takes place."* (3)

Again, he wrote, *"All pain is a break in this Vital Energy Current. All pleasure is a free full flow of it."* (4)

For Stone, all energy came from God, or Source as he called it, and must return to God, the Divine. Life was an exploration of spiritual energies in form. At the same time, while he respected mind and feeling as integral players in the dance of life, he did not see mind as the healer, in the sense that Christian Scientists of his era did, or as some New Age philosophies of our era do. The approach of mind over matter was not for him. As he wrote, *"Jesus mentioned this fact when he stated, "If a man taketh thought, can he add a cubit to his height?"* (5)

In his development of Polarity Therapy, Stone drew heavily on the Ayurvedic tradition, as well as his own experience of the human organism. Those familiar with the Ayurvedic and Vedic approach of Samkhya philosophy (see 6) will see it clearly reflected in Stone's discussion of the step-down of energy for Westerners. In Stone's description, energy first descends from the unseen into the seen manifesting as the three gunas, sattva, rajas, and tamas, as blueprints for life. He also would refer to the gunas as "principles", the air principle, fire principle, and water principle respectively. Sattva is the tree of life, the neutral blueprint underlying all existence. Rajas is the tree of nourishment, of creative outward-expanding action and service. And for Stone, tamas was described as the tree of knowledge of good and evil, the experience of materiality and the completion of the pattern in matter. (7) All three are essential for existence, and work together cooperatively to create and sustain life. He called this interlinked work of the three gunas their "triune function". (8)

Out of this blueprint for existence arise the five elements themselves, earth, water, fire, air, and space (ether). Stone based many of his treatments, and all of his approach to nutrition, on the elements. While it is evident that he was aware of the Ayurvedic concept of the five elements manifesting in the body as the three doshas (9), he never used the term "dosha" in his writing or teaching, to my knowledge. Instead, he referred exclusively to the gunas and the elements.

The name "Polarity Therapy" is based on his understanding of how the three gunas or principles manifest in form. All life and activity, including healing, is based on the interplay of these three principles. Any activity begins from the neutral still place of sattva, is carried out into the world on the active positive impulse of rajas, and returns to its source and completion via negatively charged tamas.

THE POLARITY PRINCIPLE

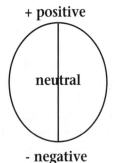

+ positive

neutral

- negative

You can carry out a simple demonstration of the gunas for yourself. Straighten up your back, let yourself get quiet and centered inside; imagine you are quite still. This clear, centered, unconditional place is sattva. Now, energetically push your hands and arms out in front of you, really throw them out there. This is rajas. Now, slowly gather your hands back toward you, letting them come to rest on your body as you complete this demonstration. This is tamas.

This interaction of the three gunas or principles creates expansion and contraction. Stone called the outwardly oriented expansive creative phase of rajas "centrifugal". The inwardly oriented contracting condensing phase of tamas he labeled "centripetal". Life is a constant balance of putting out (centrifugal motion) and receiving in (centripetal). How well we do this dance is reflected a great deal in our health and happiness. Later in his life Stone described a simple and yet quite effective way to read pulses, based on whether one needed to be expanding outward or focusing more on inward conservation. This is described more thoroughly in chapter 8. It can be an effective orientation for self-care plans.

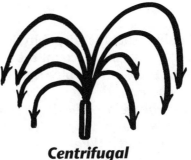

Centrifugal

CENTRIFUGAL & CENTRIPETAL

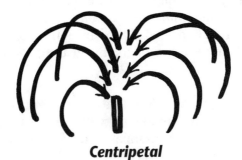

Centripetal

THE POLARITY PRINCIPLE:

POLARITY	AYURVEDA	CHINESE MED.
airy principle (neutral)	sattva (neutral)	chi
fiery principle (positive)	rajas (warm, positive, out-going)	yang (masculine)
watery principle (negative)	tamas (cool, negative, inward)	yin (feminine)

These same energies are referred to as *yang* (warm, positive) and *yin* (cool, negative) in traditional Chinese medicine and Japanese healing, and Stone construed chi as akin to the neutral force. (10) They are also expressed as the three basic postures of mind in Buddhism and Vipassana meditation.

Stone maintained that the adept physician and the astute lay person need to take into account the energy fields of the body and how these affect physical symptoms. In Dr. Stone's view, *"These subtle energy fields are facts and are not nearly as elusive as chasing thoughts and ideas around..."* (11) It was also his experience that healing energy resides in everyone: *"What healing power lies in the hands of all beings, for themselves and for others, has to be tried to be convinced by proof. It is the primal electromagnetic energy of the molecular construction of the body. It is not a mystery, nor supernatural, any more than the principle of expansion and contraction."* (12) His pioneering work with touch preceded the inception of Therapeutic Touch and many other energetic healing modalities now available.

Stone strongly maintained that Polarity principles could be used effectively in conjunction with any healing modality. While he had chosen to train as a "drugless healer", a choice that was perhaps more easily available to doctors in the early twentieth century than now, he respected his peers in Western medicine and wished they would be open to applying his methods in their practices. He believed his discoveries would benefit the application of any healing method. (13)

Stone was a radical pioneer, first describing his discoveries of the energy currents in writing in 1948. And yet, as an osteopath and chiropractor, he also oriented his work considerably around physical patterns of structural balance within the body. He wrote a great deal about how gravity, as well as the energy currents, influence structure. He was fascinated with a myriad of underlying relationships within the body, such as the connection between the sacrum of the spine and the bones of the head. As an early advocate of craniosacral therapy, he was deeply appreciative of the work of Harold Ives Magoun, D.O. (*Osteopathy in the Cranial Field*) and William Garner Sutherland, D.O., *(Teachings in the Science of Osteopathy)*. (14) And yet he made observations thirty to forty years ago that current craniosacral therapists have yet to apply: for example, he recommended working on the hands and feet as ways to balance craniosacral rhythms!

Stone advocated the use of organic foods long before most people were aware of the pesticide issue. (15) While his interests lay far more in medicine than agriculture, he applied practical mysticism regularly, for example, in his recommendations of when to harvest particular crops. (16) In this regard, one is reminded of his contemporary, Rudolph Steiner.

Stone spoke up strongly for the rights of women in the conservative post-World War II 1950's era. In sharp contrast to the existing prejudices of that time, his writings addressed women as equals in all areas. (17) (18)

Radical and mystical as he was, for many years he saw himself as a physician writing and teaching for other physicians. His seminars were "post-graduate" symposia;

many of his published works included highly technical osteopathic and chiropractic adjustments. And yet, from the outset of his practice, he was interested in what his patients could do for themselves, and self-care suggestions were sprinkled throughout his works from the late 1940's to the 1970's. (*Health Building: The Conscious Art of Living Well* was published post-humously in 1985, in an effort to address his lay audience more directly, gathering together many of his suggestions about food and Polarity Yoga.) Still, the focus of his educational efforts was aimed at physicians for many decades, with a disappointingly small response.

When Stone finally did receive public acknowledgement for his broad-ranging vision and practical healing methods, it was from unexpected quarters. In the 1960's and early 1970's he began to address as many "students of life" as he called them, as physicians, in his audiences. Young people flocked to his workshops and Randolph Stone became unexpectedly popular in his eighties. After a number of years of teaching to increasingly packed seminars, he named French-Cambodian Pierre Pannetier to succeed him in teaching the work. Stone retired in 1973 to India to be with his master, Charan Singh. Dr. Stone also continued to do work in free clinics there, as he had for decades. He died in India at the age of 91 in 1981, leaving a multitude of notes, his densely written texts, and the profession of Polarity Therapy in its infancy.

Polarity Therapy in the United States was actively preserved by communities oriented around its practices, as well as by individual students, after Randolph Stone's death. There have been ongoing struggles to clarify the intent of this dynamic work. It is still often easier to directly experience Polarity Therapy through a session than to attempt to describe it in words.

In fact, if you like, here is a simple Polarity process you can try for yourself now. It can be tried at night, when one is restless and trying to sleep, when thoughts keep rushing into one's mind. Or you can try it now, to simply calm your mind. Gently place your right hand on your forehead and your left hand on your belly. This invites the accumulated energy in your head to move downward. All you have to do is rest your hands in these spots, nothing fancy. Your right hand is acting as the active sender of energy; your left hand is the receiver. The core of your body itself acts as the neutral ground, and allows the energy to balance as it needs to do. You can maintain this position for as long as you like, or you may simply find yourself relaxing or falling asleep, into this neutral state. (If you are sitting, you are more likely to relax; lying down, to fall asleep.)

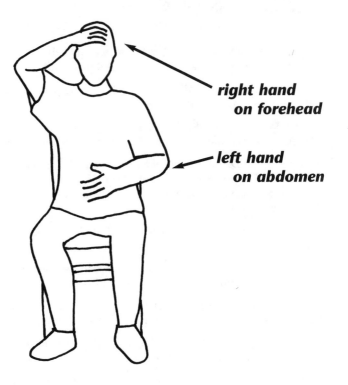

**right hand
on forehead**

**left hand
on abdomen**

A Simple Polarity Technique

If you wish to explore Polarity Therapy further, the American Polarity Therapy Association offers information, educational materials and a directory of practitioners for its members. There are centers in Europe, Mexico, Canada, Japan, and Israel as well; new programs are spreading across the globe. (See RESOURCES)

Dr. Randolph Stone was very interested in what each of us can do for ourselves, and in spreading this idea of healing energy to those who needed it. In this spirit of self-sufficiency and practicality, I offer this beginning exploration of Dr. Stone's concepts and practices. It's truly just one drop from a very wide bucket—may it be a fun and fruitful one for you!

RESOURCES IN AYURVEDA:
INTRODUCTIONS & OVERVIEWS:

Chopra, Deepak, *Perfect Health*, a readable intro to Ayurvedic Medicine from a popular Western-trained physician.

Frawley, David, *Ayurvedic Healing: A Comprehensive Guide*, much solid information for the seriously interested.

Heyn, Birgit, *Ayurvedic Medicine: The Gentle Strength of Indian Healing*, a lovely and lucid introduction from a German pharmacist.

<u>inside</u> AYURVEDA: the independent journal of Ayurvedic health care, PO Box 3021, Quincy, CA 95971-3021, USA, (530) 283-3717, journal@insideayurveda.com, a quarterly publication for Ayurvedic health care professionals.

Lad, Vasant, *Ayurveda: The Science of Self-Healing*, deceptively short book, with a lot of good information from an Ayurvedic physician.

Morrison, Judith, *The Book of Ayurveda: A Holistic Approach to Health and Longevity*, appealing well-illustrated intro.

Packard, Candis Cantin, *Pocket Guide to Ayurvedic Healing*, well-written practical intro from a Western herbalist.

Ranade, Subhash, *Natural Healing through Ayurveda*, detailed discussions from an Ayurvedic physician.

Svoboda, Robert and Arnie Lade, *Tao and Dharma: Chinese Medicine and Ayurveda*, concise and clear beginning comparison of these two systems by two skilled practitioners.

Tirtha, Swami Sada Shiva, *The Ayurvedic Encyclopedia*, a comprehensive guide to Ayurvedic healing, including herbs, foods, practices.

Yoga International is a bi-monthly journal that often integrates clear coverage of Ayurveda with yoga. RR 1, Box 407, Honesdale, PA 18431, (717) 253-4929.

AYURVEDIC ASSOCIATIONS:

American Ayurvedic Association, 719 Olde Hickory Road, Suite F, Lancaster, PA 17601, (877) 598-8830, fax: (717) 560-5614.

The National Association of Ayurvedic Medicine, 620 Cabrillo Avenue, Santa Cruz, CA 95065.

RESOURCES IN POLARITY THERAPY:
INTRODUCTIONS & OVERVIEWS:

Sills, Franklyn, *The Polarity Process: Energy as a Healing Art*, excellent and lucid overview, especially outstanding resource for bodyworkers and other therapists.

Stone, Randolph, *Health Building*, is intended as an introduction for the layperson, written in his inimitable style.

Stone, Randolph, *Polarity Therapy, volumes I & II*, is not an introduction, rather a comprehensive and wide-ranging overview of Stone's work, intended for the serious student of Polarity Therapy. Patience and something like intuition or insight are helpful qualities to bring when reading these books.

Bodary, John R., has compiled an *Index to the Polarity Writings of Dr. Randolph Stone* which is essential if you get seriously interested in Polarity Therapy; none of Stone's texts include indexes.

POLARITY THERAPY ASSOCIATIONS:

American Polarity Therapy Association (APTA), mailing address: PO Box 19858, Boulder, CO 80308; office location: 2888 Bluff St. Suite 149, Boulder, CO 80301; phone: (303) 545-2080, fax: (303) 545-2161, SATVAHQ@aol.com, maintains quarterly newsletter, bookstore, and international membership directory, including contacts for Mexico, Israel, and Europe.

Japan Polarity Therapy Association (JPTA) , address: Oguradai 4-14-12, Kitaku, Kobe, Japan 651-1211, phone & fax: 011-81-78-586-2717, email: Kpolarity@aol.com, has monthly meetings, periodic newsletter, and Polarity Therapy training coordination.

Ontario Polarity Therapy Association (OPTA), phone: 416-493-5841 (Canada) has members in Ontario and British Columbia, open to out of province members, quarterly newsletter, general meetings bi-monthly, currently developing a website.

Polarity Austria Perband Osterreich, (Austrian Polarity Therapy Association), Hollandstr. 7, A-1020 Wien, phone: 0664-5438899, fax: 0664-5476541, email: polarity-austria@gmx.at.

Polaritatsverband Deutschland (PVD), (German Polarity Therapy Association), Iris Breuert, Schottmullerstr. 7, 14167 Berlin, Germany, phone: 030-8176495, quarterly newsletter, meetings six times a year.

Polarity Verband Schweiz, (Swiss Polarity Therapy Association), phone: 061 831 25 95, fax: 061 831 38 28, regular meetings and newsletter, Polarity Therapie Zentrum Schweiz, Konradstr.14, 8005 Zurich, phone: 012731636, fax: 012731664, email: polarity@bluewin.ch, web page: www.polarity.ch.

The United Kingdom Polarity Therapy Association, Monomark House, 27 Old Gloucester Street, London WC1N 3XX England, phone: +44 (0)700 POLARITY (+44 70 07 052748) maintains a quarterly newsletter, list of accredited trainings, and international practitioner listing.

HANDS-ON POLARITY BODYWORK TEXTS:

Beaulieu, John, *Polarity Therapy Workbook*, BioSonic Enterprises, Ltd., New York, 1994.

Burger, Bruce, *Esoteric Anatomy: The Body as Consciousness*, Bruce Burger, North Atlantic Books, Berkeley, CA, 1998.

Gordon, Richard, *Your Healing Hands—The Polarity Experience*, Unity Press, Santa Cruz, CA, 1978.

Lipton, Eleanora and Alexandra Faer Bryan, *The Therapeutic Art of Polarity: An Instructional Manual for the Associate Polarity Practitioner*, Atlanta Polarity Center, 566 Pharr Road, Atlanta, GA, 30305, (404) 231-9481, ELYoga@aol.com.

Young, Phil, *The Art of Polarity Therapy: A Practitioner's Perspective*, Prism Press, Bridport, Dorset, UK, 1990.

I.

WAKING

Introducing the Elements, the Doshas and Constitutional Types.
Early Morning Routines.

MEETING DR. STONE IN HIS WRITING

Poring through Dr. Stone's writings a number of years ago, I was taken by his spiritual passion. When he said, *"There are a few things which we ourselves must do daily to keep in tune with Life and its waves of radiance, broadcasting from centers within our being and from the cosmos outside."* (1) my attention snapped to the fore. What were those things I could do?

As I searched for his answer in the passages that followed, I found myself smiling in rueful chagrin. *"Therefore, all grown-ups should consciously walk with God every hour and with every breath, and all will be given unto them. The mind becomes harsh and dominant when we forget our Creator for even one moment."* (2) High task indeed! This man was an ardent bhakti, a devotee to Spirit to the core.

Dr. Stone died in the 1980s; I never had the fortune to meet him in person. Practically though, looking at biographical photos, I can see that he must have followed his own advice. Pictures taken at sixty show a sharp, intelligent, ambitious man. Photos twenty or more years later show the same intelligence, and yet in a face tremendously softened, radiating joy. The contrast in these photos, the "before" and "after" work that Dr. Stone did with himself, is part of what keeps me exploring Polarity Therapy. It looks to me like he was on to something.

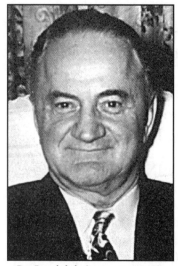
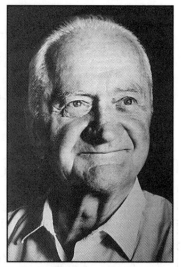

Dr. Randolph Stone at age 60.   Dr. Stone in a formal portrait taken
                                       in India when he was in his 80's.

Photographs reprinted from *Health Building*, Dr. Randolph Stone, 1985, with
permission from CRCS Publications, P.O. Box 1460, Sebastopol, CA 95472.

As we first open our eyes to a new day, anything is possible. Anything, that is, within the given limits of our bodies, hearts, minds, and spirits. In waking we arrive at our first choice point of the day, regardless of how radiant or rotten we are feeling. Do you want to take a moment or more to "tune in with Life" as Stone put it? Now is your chance.

There are many ways to "tune in", depending on your persuasion: silence, song, prayer, meditation, quiet intention, listening. Randolph Stone himself worked with the sound current, the sound of the divine, under the guidance of his spiritual teacher, Charan Singh. It is enough to remember Spirit however you choose.

THE ELEMENTS:

One way to wake up, native to this continent, is to honor the five elements and the four directions, to ground ourselves in space. The five elements are at the fundamental core of healing in both Polarity and Ayurveda. If you want, you can step outside to meet the elements, or you can discover them in whatever space you are now occupying.

The first element is space, or ether, the space around us, and the space within us. This is the space our bodies occupy physically, and the larger space we occupy energetically, when we reach out our arms and feel the energy that surrounds us. It is the space offered by our rooms, and outside, the larger space of nature. For some of us it is easier to feel the tangible space defined by our skin and bones. Others of us may find it easier to sense the larger space around us. Whatever space you notice, it can be honored, greeted. Without space, none of the other four elements can manifest.

Notice how it is possible to make contact with air. Feel the air around you: you might notice its temperature, or its smell. What are its qualities? Is it clear and sweet or thick and humid? What is it like? This is the air element currently surrounding you. It, too, can be honored and respected, if you like. You can breathe it in, and have it become a part of you, the air within.

Then as you notice warmth or cold, you can also notice light and darkness. Is the sun up? Is it shining on you? Can you feel it on your skin, on the lids of your eyes? This is fire.

If you stand in the sun, you may notice yourself begin to perspire. Here is the water element. We are close to 70% water, our physical selves. There is the moisture in our bodies, and the moisture in the air. If we are lucky, there may be water close by us, in the form of a pond or a river or an ocean or even just coming out of a faucet into a bowl we can set down close to us, as a reminder of the vitality of this element. It is water, which keeps us flowing, literally. It is the flow of feelings and the flow of the body, sweat, tears, urine, saliva. We are wet, even in the desert. An amazing package, humans. So we can honor the water within and without, if we want.

Now we get down to the nitty gritty, earth. It's the solidity of our bodies, and the ground on which we are now sitting or standing. It may be bare earth, or sand, or grass, or the floor beneath our feet. It does not usually change so fast as air or fire or water. (Hopefully! Unless we have something like an earthquake coming on.) Let yourself notice its qualities: warm, cool, hard, soft, resilient, or unyielding. It, too, can be honored, however you like.

Polarity Therapist Rose Khalsa has a traditional Native American song for the sun, which is great to sing as the sun rises. It is an ancient healing song, and goes like this:

Morning Song

Morning Sun Morning Sun,
Come my way, come my way   2 times

Come my way, come my way
Take my pain, take my pain   2 times

Take my pain, take my pain
Down below, down below   2 times

Down below, down below
Cool water down below   2 times

Give yourself time to feel all the elements all about you, the smells of the morning, the warmth of the sun, as you sing, or think about this song.

This may be all the grounding and opening you desire. Or you may find yourself wanting to greet the four directions and the above and the below as well. One way is to offer some cornmeal or tobacco in respect, to the east, and the south, and the west, and the north. And the above, and the below. You can take as long as you like to receive the nourishment of life around you, taking it in with each breath, absorbing it, releasing it with each out breath.

THE ELEMENTS AND THE SENSES:

The world nourishes us through our senses, and each sense has a resonance with an element. We perceive sound through our ears, and hearing relates to ether, space. Touch is taken in via the air element in our skin. Sight is absorbed via the fire element and the eyes. Taste is perceived when there is enough water in our mouths to activate our taste buds. The nose, via the earth element, takes in aroma, smell. Each of these elemental relationships can be used in our healing and health, working with aroma (earth), taste (water), healing views (fire), touch (air), and sound (space).

Out of the five elements springs our life experience, and the potential for healing. The elements manifest as physical states, that is, in space (as space or ether), as gas (air), temperature or energy (fire), liquid (water), and solid (earth). We see these elements every day in our own experience, as space, the wind, the sun, the rain, and the earth. In Ayurveda and Sanskrit these five great elements are known literally as *pancha mahabhutas* (*pancha* = five, *maha* = great, *bhuta* = element). The five elements are also found in Traditional Chinese Medicine and in Tibetan Buddhist Medicine. In Tibetan Buddhism, the five elements are considered alive, literally. In some Tibetan paths, they are known as the five dakinis, the consorts of the five Buddha families. (3)

THE ELEMENTS AND HEALING

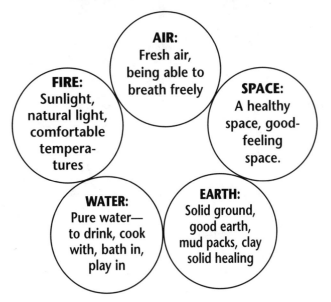

THE ELEMENTS AND POLARITY THERAPY:

I don't know that Randolph Stone ever offered cornmeal or tobacco leaves; he followed different practices in tuning in with the elements. And yet his sense was that they were vital to understand. He had an earthy, no-nonsense way of expressing how the elements operate in our bodies: *"Our body is like the house we live in; when the electric currents are on, then light and heat are available. When the water pipes are in good shape and water is pumped through them by pressure, then all the fluid requirements are solved. When the gas is turned on, then cooking and gas heating are possible. And when the drainage is not obstructed, then the sewers do not back up and no regurgitation of drainage is pocketed in any part of the basement."* (4)

Our Core:
The 3 Major Channels & the Chakras

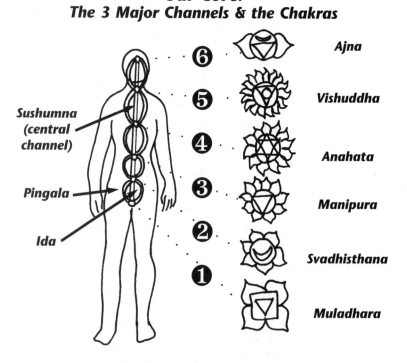

Sushumna
(central
channel)

Pingala

Ida

Ⓖ   Ajna

Ⓕ   Vishuddha

④   Anahata

❸   Manipura

❷   Svadhisthana

❶   Muladhara

In another way of looking at this, Dr. Stone was interested in mapping the elements within the body. Our core is created via sushumna, the central channel, and pingala and ida, the subtle channels weaving their way in a crisscross fashion to the right and left of sushumna, respectively. This has been represented in many cultures as the caduceus. Stone observed that each of the first five energetic chakras had a resonance with an element (see illustration, The Five Oval Fields); each of the chakras expresses a particular elemental energy. The space around these chakras creates five oval fields of healing in the human body, each also an expression of an element (see below).

The Five Oval Fields
in Relationship to the Chakras

Fire oval: the head — Sixth chakra

Ether oval: the neck — Ether chakra

Air oval: respiration — Air chakra

Earth oval: digestion & elimination — Fire chakra

Water oval: the pelvis — Water chakra

— Earth chakra

These ovals are physical fields in which energy can move. Each is created by connective tissue in the body, like the diaphragm at the chest, and the perineum at the pelvic floor. As Franklyn Sills has pointed out, "Whereas the chakras are named for the quality of energy which emanates from them, the oval fields are named for the dominant quality of movement through them." (5)

Movement, touch and thought can all be used to contact the elements in the body in Polarity Therapy. (6)

THE DOSHAS:

In Ayurveda, these elements manifest in a third way, as the doshas, which are considered three essential biological energies. The doshas are active manifestations of the elements in our bodies and in nature. The doshas are a concept unique to Ayurveda; Stone's writings do not refer to them per se. Yet an understanding of them is helpful to be able to bridge the gap of years and differing cultures, which hang between Ayurveda and Polarity. And this understanding comes in handy, in practically applying Polarity Therapy skillfully for oneself.

The three doshas, *Vata, Pitta and Kapha*, are found in every being. For a sense of their relative locations, see the illustration that follows, The Doshas.

The Doshas

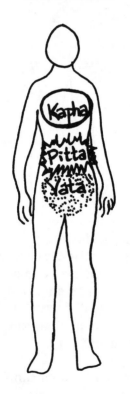

Vata arises out of air and space and finds its home in our belly, our lower abdomen, when it is happy and in balance. Vata from an Ayurvedic view is all that moves in our bodies. It is the force that moves us, from our limbs, to our nerves, to the minutest motion in a blood vessel. It is this quality of motion which keeps us flexible and adaptable, both physically and mentally. When it is out of balance, in excess, we may feel nervous or stiff or anxious or scared.

Pitta dosha, coming out of fire and water, is the fire within us, the transformative juices, our warmth, the digestive fire, the enzymes, our sharp penetrating creative intelligence. Its home, when in balance, is in the middle torso, the "fire in our bellies", the small intestine and stomach. On its own it cannot move, it relies on Vata for that. Wherever Pitta is, transformation and warmth are possible. If Pitta gets out of balance, in excess, our anger, frustration, jealousy, or inflammation can bubble to the surface faster than we intend.

Kapha arises from earth and water. It is slower, cooler, more steady than Pitta. Like Pitta, it can only move at Vata's behest. It is that quality of stability and moisture within us, our structure, solidity, immunity, endurance. Kapha's home, when it is content, is in our chest, and in the moisture in our stomachs. This protects our stomach lining from the fiery digestive fluids of Pitta. Kapha in our lungs moisturizes and tempers the air as we breathe in, helping it to acclimatize to the different environment within our bodies. Kapha throughout the body stabilizes and strengthens. When Kapha gets excessive, we may feel mired down by weight, inertia or mucus. Or we may just want to hide out. (7)

Why learn about the doshas for healing? It opens a door to many healing techniques found both in Ayurveda and Polarity. For example, Dr. Stone knew that squatting helped calm Vata (the air dosha), in one of its five forms known as "*apana*". He consciously created a squatting posture which would line up the airy energies of the body for healing. (8)

And yet students of Polarity often respond with bewilderment upon first learning about the doshas, which have not been specifically described in any of their Polarity texts. This is understandable. If you are familiar with the elemental body zones (the oval fields and chakras) of Polarity, such as water being associated with the pelvis or earth with the bowels, the doshas at first introduction can be confusing.

Here is one way to think about it. Imagine each of the Polarity oval fields is like a country (see p. 23), and the doshas are like travelers through these countries. The oval fields do not move around, they stay where they are, recognizable parts of our bodies. And yet the doshas as active biological energies are constantly moving about our bodies. Vata makes its home in the lower abdomen, which in Polarity is considered an earth oval field. Vata moves in and out of this field through the other elemental oval fields. For example, it is the energy that moves wastes out of the colon during elimination. Pitta makes its home in the mid-torso, close to the third chakra, which is related to fire in Polarity. Some similarities there. And yet from Dr. Stone's perspective, where Pitta rests is also the upper part of the earth oval field. Pitta provides the active fiery impetus for digestion in this area. Kapha makes its home in the stomach and lungs, the upper torso. In Polarity, this is the air oval field. Kapha, as an active participant in the airy lungs, moisturizes the air as it comes in, stabilizing and harmonizing this energy for the rest of the body. While the doshas can be found throughout the body, they also need to rest. Ideally, where they come home to rest is in the lower abdomen, mid-torso, and upper torso, respectively.

There are a number of ways to look at energetic anatomy. For example, in Chinese medicine, you will find the meridians. How do these relate to our picture of the doshas and the elemental fields? Meridians are like the telephone lines and roadways of the body, connecting all parts in a wide-ranging and subtle communication system. If a road is blocked or a line goes down, trouble quickly ensues.

Returning to the topic of how Ayurveda and Polarity Therapy can work together to support your health: the healthier your Kapha (earth-water dosha) is, the greater your endurance is. When Kapha is strong, it is easier to fast. When Kapha is strong, many of Polarity's dietary recommendations are easy to do. This is true, too, to a somewhat lesser extent, when Pitta (fire) is in a healthy balance. But what if your Vata dosha is out of balance? The seat of Vata is in the lower abdomen and colon. If you are a lean, thin, dry type who has been under stress, perhaps traveling a lot or simply commuting around town a bunch, many of the dietary processes Dr. Stone recommended must be done with care. Vata dosha needs to be tended astutely. Your intention is vibrant good health, not a breakdown.

THE BIOLOGICAL DOSHAS AND THEIR NEEDS

DOSHA:	NEEDS:
Vata	Safety, security
Pitta	Creative expression
Kapha	Healthy stimulation

CONNECTING WITH YOUR OWN DOSHAS

This is a simple process to begin to directly experience the biological energies of the doshas for yourself. Let yourself get in a comfortable position: sitting is easiest for this one. You will be putting your hands on the front and back sides of your body, centering around the home site of each dosha. You can start with your right palm resting on your lower abdomen, the home of Vata, with your left hand directly behind it, posterior, on your back. Sit with your eyes closed and take a few deep breaths at whatever pace you like, to settle in. Your intention in this process is simply to connect with Vata, get a sense of how it is feeling in this moment. Does the area feel warm or cool, slow or active? Notice also how your hands feel: warm, or cool, steady, or a little trembly?...Any of these responses would be normal, and lets you know a little more about your personal relationship with this dosha. When you've spent as much time information-gathering with Vata as you want, take a break to jot down your impressions.

Homes of the Doshas

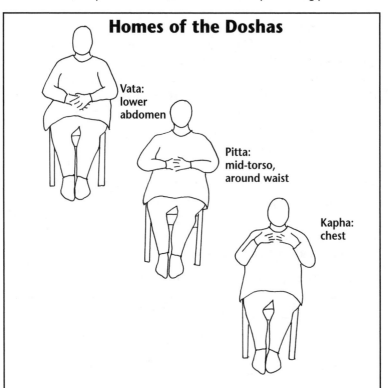

Vata:
lower
abdomen

Pitta:
mid-torso,
around waist

Kapha:
chest

When you're ready, continue on with Pitta. The process is the same: your clear intention is to connect with Pitta now. Placing your hands front to back just above your waist and navel, allow yourself to notice what you feel. Does the area feel energized or slow? What kind of a feeling do you get from this area? Again, when you feel complete with this, relax and write down a few notes about what you discovered.

Continue on with Kapha, in the chest. If there was one word or phrase to describe how this area feels, what would it be? Write down your impressions, again noting whether it feels cool or warm, strong or weak, on the surface or submerged. When you are done with exploring all three areas, which might take fifteen minutes or more, stretch and take a break. If you're doing this with a friend or in a group, now is a good time to share your observations with one another.

Mantra & Dosha

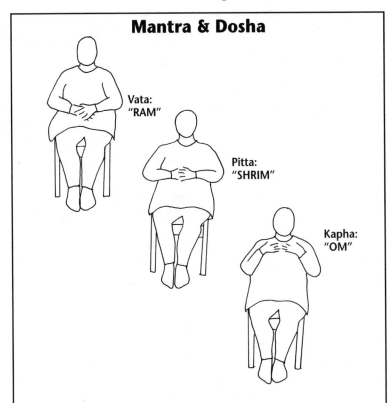

Vata: "RAM"

Pitta: "SHRIM"

Kapha: "OM"

In the ancient Ayurvedic texts it was said that problems with illness or our bodies arose when one or more of the three doshas wandered from their home sites. We have just connected with these home zones in the previous process. Vata's home is the lower abdomen, Pitta's the mid-torso just above the navel, and Kapha's is in the chest.

Traditionally, mantra, or healing sound has been used to invite the doshas back home. There are many mantras that can be used for this purpose, and yet I'd like to keep us simple here. OM is helpful for calming Kapha. SHRIM (shreem) soothes Pitta well. RAM tonifies and settles Vata.

In this modern adaptation of Ayurvedic self-healing, as you put your hands on the home of Vata in the lower abdomen, you can tone RAM. As you touch your Pitta zone, around your middle, you can sing SHRIM. And as you bring your hands up to your chest to invite Kapha home, you can chant OM. Simple. Try it.

If you have tried this and like it, you can reverse the order, starting with Kapha and the chest, then moving down to Pitta mid-torso, then further down to Vata in the lower abdomen, OM, SHRIM, RAM. All three syllables can be sung together, one after another, three or four times or more, gently touching each zone in turn, sending love and healing intent as you sing. This is one safe and pleasurable way to begin to balance your own doshas.

THE DIRECTIONAL FLOW OF ENERGY IN THE ELEMENTS:

Each of the elements has a characteristic way it tends to flow. Air and fire tend to flow upward (think of how hot air rises toward the ceiling in a room). Earth and water naturally gravitate downward (imagine a creek flowing down hill, or a clod of dirt falling to the ground). Ether, the space element, holds space neutrally, with no particular directional movement.

Directional Flow of the Elements

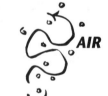 AIR

FIRE

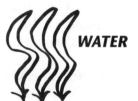 WATER

EARTH

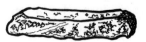

When air or fire are activated or out of balance, many thoughts or feelings may rush upward into our minds. When water or earth predominate, our energy may hide out below out belts, so to speak, or even in our toes. This will be a wild concept for some, and perfectly natural for others, depending on your experience and cultural expectations. It can prove quite useful in helping yourself. If you did the opening relaxation in the introduction about Polarity Therapy, you were using directional healing in that process. Your right hand on the head was inviting all the upward rushing mental energy to begin to move downward, to settle and ground. Doing this process, you might have felt less "up in the air".

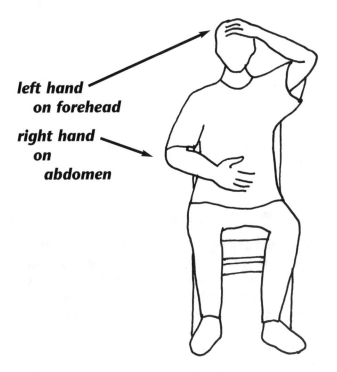

left hand on forehead

right hand on abdomen

Another Simple Polarity Technique

What if you were to reverse this process, put your right hand on your belly and your left on your forehead? From a Polarity Therapy perspective, this would encourage energy to move upward. Your right hand sends the energy from the abdomen, your left hand receives it up at your head. This kind of hold would be useful if you were feeling stuck and not sure what your "gut" feeling about something was. You can invite the information hidden below your belt into your mind. This directional flow of energy can feel particularly good to people who have a fair amount of earth or water in their make-ups. For more about how Dr. Stone perceived the directions of the elements, see (9).

SOME SIMPLE WORK WITH THE DOSHAS: BODYWORK

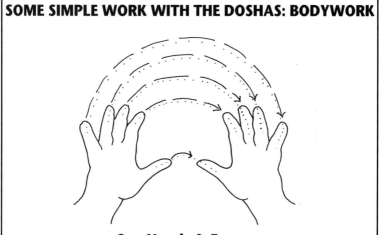

Our Hands & Energy

Once you have an opening sense of the doshas, you have the option to work with them further, using principles of Polarity Therapy. For most people, our right hand has the potential to send energy, while the left hand is especially good for receiving energy. Either hand can be used for these two functions, yet for most people, energy is easiest to experience if the right hand is used to send out energy, the left to receive it. You can use your hands in a variety of ways. For example, if your Vata zone felt a little shaky and tenuous, you might simply place both hands on the lower abdomen and send love and comfort there.

In Ayurveda, the doshas are found everywhere in the body, yet they each have these home sites where they reside. If they are expelled from their homes, or wander, the sensations can be most uncomfortable. For example, lower abdominal surgery often disrupts Vata. Something like a hysterectomy can be very difficult for Vata's normal balance. In a situation such as this, the energy can be invited back home, to its original zone. Sometimes this occurs quickly; or it can take a number of steady invitations over weeks, to really bring the biological energy back into its center. When it does get "home", there can be a sense of deep relief.

In one self-care group of which I am a part, we did the CONNECTING WITH THE DOSHAS process described earlier. One participant reported that she had been having troubles with indigestion the last few days, not a usual experience for her. When she checked in with her doshas, it felt like Pitta was irritated and extending up into the chest, into Kapha's zone. When we began to work with our own doshas, she chose to put her right hand on her chest and her left hand on Pitta's zone in the mid-torso, inviting the errant fiery energy back home. Her digestion felt much better with just ten minutes of this kind of work.

For some other examples: an overly active mind is a common challenge. From an Ayurvedic perspective, too much Vata is racing up into our heads! You can place your right hand on your forehead and your left on your lower abdomen, to invite the airy Vata mental energy downward. Or, for a different example, perhaps there is congestion, even water retention, in your feet and ankles. You can place your right hand on an ankle or your toes, your left on your heart or chest, inviting balance back in, as Kapha returns home. (This is no substitute for a visit to the cardiologist, you understand.) These are not instant cures for edema or hyperactive mind, yet you are likely to feel better, and you are letting your body know it is okay to rebalance in a healthy way.

> These same principles can be used in doing bodywork with another person.
>
> If you are an experienced body worker, an obvious question comes up: How do you know you are connecting with the doshas and not muscle or membrane or the elemental ovals of Polarity, or what? The key here is intention. You are tuning your radio station, so to speak, to receive the "doshas" channel, and not something else. It sounds surprisingly simple, yet it can work quite effectively.

ABOUT MANTRA AND HEALING:

When we are using something as ephemeral as mantra, it is easy to question its efficacy, although the healing power of sound has been well documented for years. I had an experience with the silent use of mantra many years ago that gave me pause.

About twenty years ago I was working a fair amount with death and dying and folks in hospice. One woman I had been sent to visit at home became a good friend, and we saw one another often. She was not an official hospice patient, and was receiving general home care from our agency. Lee had had lung cancer twice already and she confided in me that she sensed that if it recurred a third time, in her bone, that was it for her. She lived alone, and was a very independent type of person. She had several good friends in our town, yet her family lived far away. We shared meals and I brought her little goodies, healthy ones, hoping to help her.

One night, at home in my apartment, I lay dreaming that there was a wolf at the door. The dream was interrupted by a phone call; it was 3:00 in the morning. The hospital was calling. Lee had been admitted earlier that day; she was in a lot of pain. Could I come?

When I got there, Lee was clear, conscious, focused most on breathing and writhing. Between her and the nurse I got the basics: the cancer had reoccurred, it was in her bone, and she was now in a dying process. She was conscious and determined to live until the morning, when a lawyer was scheduled to come help her work out her will, which held many emotional complications.

As I sat there with her, her pain became more than I could bear. I asked her if she needed more morphine. She'd had the maximum, she said. It got worse, I talked with the nurse. She said: "If we give her any more morphine, it could kill her." I thought, well, isn't that what Lee is doing anyway? But Lee herself was adamant: she had to make it to 8:30 a.m., when the lawyer was due to come. It got worse, if such a thing was possible. I realized that I might be able to get hold of some extra morphine from my work through another hospice program. But Lee was again adamant: the pain was awful, and she needed to stay alive. I had seen people stay in similar states for days, even a week, and so that certainly seemed possible to me. First off I needed to honor Lee's choices. Yet I also had to deal with my own agony, as I silently bathed her. She had gotten to a place where conversation was not welcome, and yet the coolness of the washcloth helped her.

As I struggled with myself, the question came to me: "What do I believe in, drugs or God?" (Well obviously, drugs, but I wasn't getting far with those.) I began to work with mantra, a very simple one my teacher used. With every breath I repeated to myself, "RAM". I did it silently so as not to disturb Lee. It was about 5:15 to 5:30 a.m. by this time, and Lee's mantra was, literally, "AWFUL". We did our mantras together, she with every out breath, me silently. I said nothing, as Lee was still in no mood for conversation. In desperation, I just kept repeating RAM to myself. In a half an hour Lee had quieted, her breathing calmed, and she moved into a profoundly peaceful state. Another half hour or so, and she passed—in deep peace.

I was stunned and grateful. How could this be? She was out of her pain and had died in peace. I had not expected this. Many complications lay ahead with the family and the will, yet I could tell them in all honesty she had died in peace.

I have been at a few births, and more deaths. My impression from being with friends dying is that it looks a lot like birth: there is a labor, sometimes short, sometimes long, there is a breath—and then it all changes, we go. For me with Lee, I had never seen someone die so fast or go from such an extreme state of pain to one of peace.

Which is all to say, perhaps mantra could help with that headache or tummy pain, yes?

OTHER SUPPORTS:

There are many other Ayurvedic practices to calm the doshas. One comforting one is *abhyanga*, oil massage, which is specifically designed to calm Vata, so that a person can cleanse without getting uncomfortably shaky or sore. A practice like abhyanga, combined with Ayurvedic or Polarity purifying processes, can make cleansing a lot easier to do. There is more information about abhyanga further on in this chapter.

CONSTITUTIONAL TYPES:

Each of us has all three doshas; for good health, like the elements, we need them all to flourish, whether we are consciously aware of them or not. (See chart: THE FIVE ELEMENTS AND THE CONSTITUTIONS). Yet each of us is an individual, with a slightly different balance of the elements and the doshas inside. This difference is manifested in our lifelong constitution and essential nature, what in Polarity is called our constitutional type, and in Ayurveda, our *prakruti*. Our constitutional type is reflected in areas like our basic body build, our temperament, our hair color, and our endurance.

The Five Elements and the Constitutions

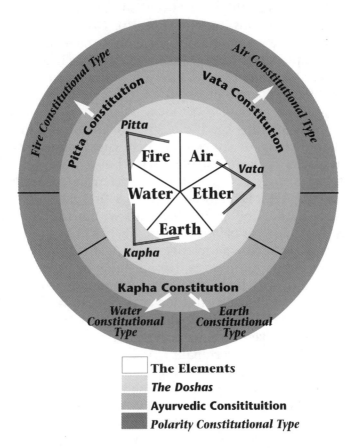

All of these can change, especially in this day and age, and when they do, it is known in Ayurveda as our *vikruti* or current imbalance. Underneath the current imbalance or appearance of things, our innate birth tendencies remain. The chunky kid of childhood hides under the svelte beauty of adulthood. The fiery redhead may now be a young bleached blond with black and green streaks running through his hair, and yet he still struggles with his temper as he negotiates his skate board across the town square. The skinny bespeckled ten-year-old may have grown into a man who lifts weight, plays football, and looks pretty buff. Yet under that solid earthy appearance may still lurk the worries and insecurities of the airy Vata constitution.

When we work with ourselves or others, it's helpful to acknowledge this duality: the current condition (vikruti) and the underlying constitution (prakruti). Otherwise we risk insulting ourselves or others. For example, many airy types reside in apparently large, solid, earthy-looking bodies. This can occur for many reasons: safety, protection, and security being a few of them.

In Ayurveda, this specific balance of the doshas in any given individual is known as their constitutional type. Perhaps you've heard someone say, "I'm a Vata." or "My husband is so Pitta." Here they are referring to constitutional type. Yet it is important to realize that each of us has all three doshas and all five elements within us. When all three doshas are in balance we are likely to feel healthiest and most centered. The relative balance of the doshas and elements shows up in areas like our body build, or in our emotional approach to life. So for example, someone with Vata strong in their constitution may tend to be lean and mentally flexible. Whereas someone with Pitta predominant is more likely to have a medium build and a more assertive or leading personality. A Kapha could be stocky, patient, more steady in applying themselves to a task than their Pitta or Vata friends. Yet how each of us manifests these is unique to us. We are not neat tidy cookie cutter shapes, coming in just three flavors. These concepts can be used to promote healing in many powerful ways. (10)

Both Polarity Therapy and Ayurveda acknowledge these unique differences in our constitutions. If you are familiar with Polarity, yet not Ayurveda, you can access a lot of knowledge from the ancient texts by realizing that air types are synonymous with Vata types, fire types with Pitta types, and earth and water types both are found in Kapha type.

In Ayurveda, the three primary constitutional types are: Vata (air-ether), Pitta (fire-water), and Kapha (earth-water) In Polarity, Stone differentiated the constitutional types further, making four types. When reading Ayurvedic or Polarity literature, it is fairly easy to make the transition between these groupings. Vata constitution is identical to Polarity's air constitutional type; Pitta constitution is the same as Polarity's fire type. Kapha, Dr. Stone differentiated into two distinct types, the Polarity water type and the Polarity earth type. At first this was confusing to me, I didn't understand the point he was making. However, it is a good one.

There is a practical difference between the Polarity water type and the Polarity earth type, in terms of how you work with yourself and others. A watery type is more changeable, shifting their thoughts and ideas with the flow of their feelings. They may look solid, yet they will often have a changeable eating style, depending on how they feel. They could have challenges with water retention, or fluid flow in their bodies. This Polarity water type would be known as one kind of Kapha in Ayurveda.

The earth type, still known as a Kapha in Ayurveda, is quite different. They feel most comfortable with steady habits and routines. They do not see themselves as changeable, and they probably aren't. In fact, they are the least likely of the four types to spontaneously embrace a new lifestyle plan suddenly. Change does not come easily to the Polarity earth type. However, they will stick with a program once they are committed to it, and are less easily swayed by changes in feeling than the water type.

CONSTITUTIONAL TYPES

POLARITY	AYURVEDA	Brief Description
air type	Vata	Small boned, often long fingers or toes, can be lean, with active mind. Mentally flexible.
fire type	Pitta	Medium boned, assertive nature, strong initiative. May have fair or ruddy complexion with reddish or light hair.
water type	Kapha	Solid or large boned, tendency to hold water or feelings, changeable emotionally. Patient with others.
earth type	Kapha	Solid or large-boned, solid neck, strong habits, changes slowly both mentally and emotionally. Strong endurance, usually patient with others.

Where I live here in northern New Mexico, we use irrigation ditches called acequias. The water that flows through the ditch to nourish the plants is like the water type, nurturing, changeable, sometimes here, sometimes not. The embankments that hold the water to its flow are like the earth type, steady, unchanging, keeping the water flowing within safe limits. Without earth, the water could flood all over. Without water, the earth can become dry and hard. Each type is important in the dance of life. We will be talking more about each type and their needs as we go on.

EARLY MORNING ROUTINES:

Enough for overview! You're awake, you've gotten out of bed, you are heading for the bathroom. (Note: While I leap here from bed to bathroom, not all of us are in a position to do this so blithely. If you have back problems, or use a wheel chair, just to name a couple of circumstances, movement and stretching may be your first items of the day, and may take place in bed.)

The first thing Randolph Stone recommended in a morning routine was a liver-flush, a concoction of fresh lemon and orange juice to enliven a sluggish liver. Depending on your preferences, you may want to pause in the bathroom as part of your self-care. Or you may head straight for the kitchen and the lemon juice cleanse (see LIVER FLUSH, chapter 6).

Ayurveda, which Dr. Stone drew on strongly in his development of Polarity, is famed for its daily rituals and routines to enhance well being. Two very useful routines that can be integrated into any self-care plan are *abhyanga* (oil massage) and *neti* and *nasya* (nasal cleansing). A third is tongue scraping. While the first two have exotic names and the last sounds potentially lethal, all three are actually pretty simple, painless and straightforward to do.

TONGUE CLEANING

To start with your tongue, if you're inclined: tongue scraping is easy to do before brushing your teeth in the morning. You can use a metal spoon or a horseshoe shaped tongue scraper made especially for the purpose (the $3 or $4 variety work just as well as those marketed for $20. In fact, they appear to be identical). You gently scrape any accumulated coat off your tongue; usually it is thickest toward the back. This has a number of purposes: it clears the tongue and freshens the breath. More importantly for health, it sends messages to the gut via the nerves that you are ready to clear out the colon, a good prelude to elimination or any kind of gastro-intestinal cleansing. A dozen strokes from back to front are usually plenty.

ABHYANGA: OIL MASSAGE

The reason for *abhyanga* is simple, from an Ayurvedic point of view. Abhyanga is especially calming to Vata and airy types. Excess Vata, air dosha, accumulates on the skin. When we massage ourselves with oil, this excess air—and concomitant dryness and nervous energy—calm down. Dawn and dusk are considered powerful transition points in the day, and practices done at these times gain potency. So oil massage done when we first get up, before we take a shower or bath, calms Vata very well. This strengthens not only the skin, but also muscle, concentration, and overall stability. The yogis have known this for centuries. If we are anxious, nervous, forgetful, stiff, achy, constipated, or twitchy, abhyanga is useful. Conversely, if we are in the middle of a cleanse and start to notice these signs, it is an indication that Vata is out of balance and needs immediate help. Dr. Stone often advocated oil massage, especially after a bath. Whether you choose to do it before the bath or after is a matter of personal choice. You might try a month each way and see which suits you best. If you are doing Dr. Stone's baking soda rub (see below), it makes most sense to do the soda rub first, in the shower, and follow with the oil rub, as Dr. Stone called it. Both can feel very good.

For years I was told about the benefits of abhyanga. And I would do it sporadically (maybe I am back to sporadic as you read this). There are lots of reasons to skip abhyanga: you're in a hurry, the bathroom's too cold, you don't want to get all oily, etc. However, if you are an airy or fiery type and can persuade yourself to do it regularly, you are likely to be rewarded for your steady efforts. It calms and strengthens one.

There is a wide variety of oils or ghee you can use. The simpler and purer they are, the better. If you want to get fancy, you can make your own medicated oils or ghees or purchase them. Right now I'm using a homemade salve to nourish the bones which I like a lot (see Appendix: PERSONAL SELF-CARE RECIPES). However, simple sesame oil, extra virgin olive oil, sweet almond oil, coconut butter, or castor oil work fine. Sesame and olive oil are most easily found in organic forms, to minimize toxic chemicals.

Traditionally one uses long strokes, covering the whole body generously and lovingly in oil from top to toe. Earthy and watery types may be happy with much smaller amounts of oils, or even dusting dry herbal powders on oneself instead. You can make a production of it, or be finished with the whole process in less than five minutes, depending on your inclination. A plastic squeegee bottle waiting on the bathroom counter helps. You can squirt some oil on your hands in controllable amounts, smooth it on one area, then go on to the next. If you look like a drowned rat with oil on your hair, you might skip your head and just do your neck and face and the rest of your body. (If you like, you can make up for this by periodically dousing your head with oil before bed and letting it soak in well all night, with your pillow protected by an old towel. Abhyanga to the head is quite valued in Ayurveda.)

After you've taken a few minutes to oil yourself up, you can then step into a warm shower or bath and let the oil percolate inward. By the time you step out, you are likely to feel well moisturized, yet not greasy, with a minimum of oil to get on your clean bath towel. But what if you are an earthy or watery type? All this oil may sound disgusting. A light dusting of the herb *brahmi* (powdered gotu kola) between your palms and all over your body may feel more stimulating and appropriate. Or again, check out Dr. Stone's baking soda rub, otherwise known as salt glow.

Alternatively, abhyanga can be done before bed. In either case, your muscles can feel as relaxed as if they themselves were a comfy pair of pajamas.

DR. STONE'S BAKING SODA RUB

Dr. Stone used baking soda and salt on a wet washcloth to clear the skin of sticky residues and open the pores. This cleansing is quite easy to do. With a container of baking soda and one of sea salt waiting for you on the tub side, step into the bathtub and get your washcloth wet with a little soap on it (some might want to skip the soap entirely, if their skin is quite dry). Then pour two tablespoons of baking soda directly on to your washcloth, followed by one tablespoon of salt. Rub this "salt glow" all over your body, including your face and neck. As Stone says, "(it) *has the soothing effect of bathing in the ocean."* Rinse yourself well with warm water, followed by a vigorous cool rinse *"for about fifteen minutes"* (11), letting the water hit your back and spine. This closes the pores and strengthens your immunity. Dr. Stone's oil rub is done before drying off. Using just a little pure oil in your hands, rub it well into your whole body. Vigorously dry off whatever moisture is left with a bath towel. If you want to use more soda and salt, that's fine; Stone often recommended they be used in this two to one proportion, but he recommended other proportions on occasion as well. He was more interested in people doing it in general than following rigorous proportions.

The baking soda rub is likely to feel especially invigorating to fiery, watery, and earthy types. Airy types may find that regular use is drying for their skin.

Cleansing with a Neti Pot

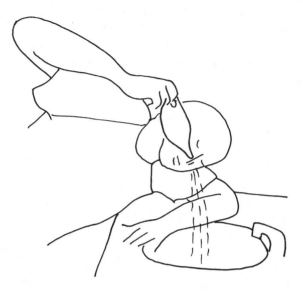

NETI AND NASYA:
(sounds like two aging aunts, yes?)

Neti and nasya, two forms of nasal cleansing, can be more of a stretch culturally. Yet they are both simple and can feel quite good when you're done. Because both gently cleanse the sinuses, they can relieve blockages, including sinusitis, headaches, chronically stuffy nose, and held-in feelings. Both can be done as needed, or as often as once a day. Neti is nasal cleansing with a water solution; nasya cleanses or builds using herbs in an oil base. In my area, where it is very dry, doing neti twice a week is considered enough, as the daily drying effect of the water on the nose could be more than is needed. Doing neti first thing in the morning, say before you brush your teeth, works well. While traditionally in Ayurveda a neti pot is used (see RESOURCES), one Polarity teacher of mine uses saline solution in a re-usable little squeegee bottle. Whatever is your pleasure.

Neti pots look like small ceramic teapots, and literally act like that too. You can put a cup of R.O.-purified water on to boil when you first get up, then pour the boiled water into a heat-proof Pyrex measuring cup with a pinch of sea salt. (R.O. water is water that has been purified by a reverse osmolarity process, hence the initials. It is commonly found in supermarkets in special dispenser stations for purified water here in the United States. Other sorts of pure water can also be used, such as distilled, if the water hasn't sat so long in a plastic bottle as to take up substantial quantities of plastic.) Let the saline solution sit on the bathroom counter while you are taking your shower. It can cool to a good temperature by the time you step out. The water should be comfortably warm to the touch. The process is easier if you blow your nose before you begin.

Pour half a cup of the water into your pot and slowly slowly gently tip your head over the bathroom sink, the tip of the neti pot at one nostril, as if you were about to pour tea in your nose. Strange, yes, but cheaper than antihistamines, and quite safe. Slowly pour all this first saline solution into whichever nostril you are cleansing. After a moment or two, the solution will start dribbling out your other nostril into the sink, as it passes through your nasal cavity. Finally you will have poured it all in, in a few moments, and it will all have dribbled out the other nostril (if it comes down your throat, lean forward a little until it is coming through your nose instead). It will probably feel good to blow your nose or spit, to clear any excess out. Then you can do the other side in the same way. Voila! Clear sinuses!

This is also an effective protective technique if you feel you may be coming down with a cold. If you like, gently massaging a little sesame oil or ghee into your clean nostrils will give extra protection to these membranes.

Nasya is done with special oil preparations. These can be used daily as part of a self-care program (for example, brahmi oil is used to strengthen the memory), or as part of a special series of Ayurvedic cleansings known as Pancha Karma.

If you find yourself enjoying these morning routines, there are many fine self-care techniques offered in *Ayurvedic Beauty Care* by Melanie Sachs, including recipes for massage lotions and shampoos, simple facials, and effective body-work (see RESOURCES).

————•————

CHAPTER SYNOPSIS:

WAKING:

Do you want to:

remember the sacred?

greet the sun and the elements?

brush your teeth?

scratch your chin?

scrape your tongue?

wash your face?

do abhyanga (oil massage) before a shower?

blow your nose or do nasya?

eliminate?
or

do none of the above: just keep sleeping?

RESOURCES IN WAKING:
BOOKS:

Dr. Stone, *Health-Building*, CRCS Press, entire.

Arewa, Caroline Shola, *Opening to Spirit: Contacting the Healing Power of the Chakras & Honouring African Spirituality*, beautiful book with a strong focus on the chakras, with Polarity techniques.

Chakravarti, Sree, *A Healer's Journey*, see chapter 28, Using Sound to Heal, p. 221-223.

Gordon, Richard, *Your Healing Hands*, an excellent intro to using your hands therapeutically.

Sachs, Melanie, *Ayurvedic Beauty Care*, with recipes for massage oils.

Svoboda, Robert, *Prakriti: Your Ayurvedic Constitution*, well-written book about the Ayurvedic concept of constitution.

Morningstar, Amadea and Urmila Desai, *The Ayurvedic Cookbook*, pages 8-20, has specific information about constitutional types.

Tiwari, Maya, *Ayurveda: A Life of Balance*, explores Ayurveda and constitution, working with everyday processes as spiritual practice.

Verma, Vinod, *Ayurveda: A Way of Life*, introduces many practical self-care methods.

ELEMENTAL RETREATS, POLARITY TRAININGS IN NATURE:

This is a partial listing: please contact the American Polarity Therapy Association for updated information. Also, APTA holds its national conference each year in late June in nature, in varying locales across the country, (303) 545-2080, email: SATVAHQ@aol.com.

Center for World Indigenous Studies, offers both training and renewal retreats in the jungles of Mexico; its intent is to advance cooperation and consent between nations. It also offers writer's independent retreats (by arrangement), trainings in traditional medicine, energy medicine, and women's health under the direction of Leslie Korn, PhD, MPH, RPP. There are opportunities for community service in village life, internships, in Xipe Totec, Yelapa, Mexico. For more information, contact Registrar, PMB 214, 1001 Cooper Point Rd SW #140, Olympia, WA 98502-1107 (USA), Joyce at (360) 754-1990, joyce@cwis.org, web page: www.cwis.org.

EarthWise Retreat, is held mid-winter at Ghost Ranch, New Mexico, in beautiful, high mountain-desert country, for relaxation, learning and healing. Trainings in Polarity, yoga, herbs, nutrition in relaxed setting. Sweat lodge. Contact Damon Fazio, ND, RPP, LMT, Earth Wise Therapy, 1612 Hendola Dr. NE, Albuquerque, NM 87110, (505) 294-4505, email: dafaz@earthlink.net.

Jacobs, Jeffrey, DOM, RPP, International Wellness Inc, New York, NY, phone: (917) 933-9720, email: JHJAKE1@aol.com, offers an annual 6 day Polarity retreat on the big island of Hawaii. There are also plans to do retreats in Japan, in monastery/temple setting.

Kolman, Moksha Sharon, RPP, Center for Natural Healing, no retreats yet, just vibrant, clear Polarity trainings with a strong focus on the elements, Timberlake, NC, (336) 364-3114.

The Polarity Center and Shamanic Studies, has a yearly program called The Shaman's Circle, that meets monthly in a beautiful, quiet retreat center in the mountains of Sugarloaf, in Mt. Airy, Maryland. It offers in-depth training in Shamanism with an emphasis on Native American spirituality and Tibetan Shamanism. Contact Rose Khalsa, RPP, 9 Philadelphia Ave, Tacoma Park, MD, 20912, (301) 891-1599, e-mail: rosediana@erols.com, web page: www.erols.com/rosediana.

Tree of Life Polarity Center, Janice Marie, Durand, RPP, heart-felt Polarity trainings and retreats in nature, PO Box 281, Saxapahaw, NC 27340 (near Raleigh-Durham), (336) 376-8186, email: jmdchi@mindspring.com.

Wellness Professionals, offer energetic learning experiences in beautiful natural environments. Workshops are organized around a topic such as Healthcare for the Nervous System, Energetic Spa Treatments, or Working with Trauma, with plenty of time to relax and play. Locations include 100 acre woodlands and country house with private lake in Ohio, and ocean view retreats on Kauai, Hawaii's "Garden Island". Contact: Gary Peterson, RPP, 2475 Juniper Ave., Boulder, CO 80304, (303)541-9893, email: satvagp@earthlink.net.

See also: Polarity Cleansing Retreats in Nature, under RESOURCES, chapter 6, for more listings.

Supplies:

Banyan Trading Company, wholesale to health practitioners. Good source for reasonably priced tongue scrapers, as well as simple oils such as sesame or medicated oils, e.g., ashwaganda-bala oil, a tonic oil which strengthens muscles and nerves, 1 (800) 953-6424, www.banyantrading.com, retail: www.banyanbotanicals.com.

Lotus Light and Lotus Brands, for a wide array of books and self-care products related to Ayurveda and healing.

Internatural
33719 116th St.
Twin Lakes, WI 53181 USA
800-643 4221 (toll free order line)
262-889 8581 (office phone)
262-889 8591 (fax)
E-mail: internatural@lotuspress.com
Website: www.internatural.com
Retail mail order and internet reseller of Ayurvedic products, essential oils, herbs, spices, supplements, herbal remedies, incense, books and other supplies.

Lotus Brands, Inc.
P. O. Box 325
Twin Lakes, WI 53181 USA
Ph: 262-889-8561
Fax: 262-889-8591
E-mail: lotusbrands@lotuspress.com
Website: www.lotusbrands.com
Manufacturer and distributor of natural personal care and herbal products, massage oils, essential oils, incense, aromatherapy items, dietary supplements and herbs.

Lotus Light Enterprises
P. O. Box 1008
Silver Lake, WI 53170 USA
800-548 3824 (toll free order line)
262-889 8501 (office phone)
262-889 8591 (fax)
E-mail: lotuslight@lotuspress.com
Website: www.lotuslight.com
Wholesale distributor of essential oils, herbs, spices, supplements, herbal remedies, incense, books and other supplies. Must supply resale certificate number or practitioner license to obtain catalog of more than 10,000 items.

Real Goods: neti pots and other sustainable items, 200 Clara Avenue, Ukiah, CA 95482-4004, (800) 762-7325, www.realgoods.com.

The Himalayan Publishers, Dept. YIMN, RR1 Box 405, Honesdale, PA 18431, (800) 822-4547, fax (717) 253-9078, neti pots and other supplies for yoga.

II.

MOVEMENT

Understanding the Three Energy Currents and the Gunas.

"The three gunas are everywhere the attributes of matter and motion, as positive (+), negative (-), and neuter (0). Everywhere is life in motion... " STONE, HEALTH BUILDING, P. 15

"The Wireless Energy Currents of Polarity in the body are beneficially affected as one gently and gracefully wiggles into the postures." STONE, HEALTH BUILDING, P. 98

POLARITY AND MOVEMENT:

The whole focus of Polarity Therapy is to get energy moving. Its founder declared the free flow of energy *"the primal factor in health and beauty"*. (1) One of the best ways to free up your energy is to get yourself moving in ways you like. The purpose of movement here is self-exploration, healing and a direct experience of energy.

Dr. Stone came up with a whole series of exercises known as Polarity Yoga to stimulate the free flow of energy in the body. These feel great early in the morning to clear out the kinks and prepare oneself for meditation, or they can be done late at night, before retiring. Again, the focus of Polarity Yoga is to be able to directly experience your energy currents rather than build or develop muscle. As you become adept at moving with these energies, you may find yourself becoming more physically flexible or strong as well. And yet it is the free flow of energy that is the aim, rather than muscle.

In another approach, Charmaine Lee, a Polarity Therapist and professional dancer centered in the Washington D.C. area, has developed a subtle, sophisticated and fun way to dance one's way to health. Charmaine evolved SynergyDance as a way of caring for herself when she found herself isolated in an area where no other Polarity Therapists lived. She wanted to activate the energy currents that Stone described in his books. As she says, "I moved the physical body in the energy patterns (of the three currents), which gave rise to the subtle energy moving me."(2) Working with these patterns of movement is like giving oneself a Polarity Therapy session. They stimulate circulation to needed areas, free up the flow of energy in the body, and simply feel good. Some of Charmaine's inspired techniques are presented in the pages that follow; there is more information about SynergyDance in the RESOURCES section at the end of this chapter.

As Lee suggests, the energy of the currents can be traced directly on your own. I have done this with a series of movements rather like Chi Gung or Tai Chi, called Three Current Chi Gung. These can be a powerful way to access the healing energy of the currents. In Three Current Chi Gung, you activate the energy of your body by running your hands over the pathways of the currents. Following the three specific patterns of the currents can be an excellent warm-up for Polarity Yoga or SynergyDance. It can also be done on its own to stimulate healing.

THE THREE ENERGY CURRENTS:

As discussed in the introductory chapters, Randolph Stone described currents of life force, which flow through and around our bodies. These currents arise out of the chakras. While the chakras are an integral part of ancient Yoga and Ayurveda, Stone's work with the currents flowing from the chakras is his unique contribution to healing. It is what makes Polarity Therapy more than just a synthesis of Western naturopathy, Ayurveda, and Chinese Medicine concepts. Stone worked with three patterns: the transverse current, the spiral current, and the long line currents in a myriad of ways, using a variety of bodywork and movement techniques to access their healing potentials. He likened his identification of these currents to other discoveries related to energy, such as atomic physics. His hope was that, as modern physics and research into the atom had opened a new vision of the underlying energy fields within matter, physicians could do the same in their work with patients. He imagined medicine expanding beyond its reliance on physical measures into an understanding and application of the energy fields that activate each person. (3)

Clearly, Stone was not the first to conceive of this reality. One thinks about poet Walt Whitman writing in *Leaves of Grass* in the 1800's, "*I sing the body electric...*" Yet Randolph Stone explored and described "the body electric" more thoroughly than anyone before him. He perceived that the three currents were vehicles for the movement of prana or chi; sometimes calling them "Prana Currents". (4)

The currents are a way to enhance vitality and speed healing. They can be accessed through touch, movement, and thought. With practice, they can be sensed with the hands and assessed visually in how we move.

Each of the currents has a characteristic path and motion. And each current is an expression of a particular quality of mind and energy, a way of being. These qualities or principles have a resonance with the mental qualities known in Ayurveda as *gunas*. Stone retained this same term in his writing about Polarity Therapy, though he would also call these qualities "principles". Gunas or principles, the concept is the same: spirit manifests in mind, which then manifests in form, in three ways. There is balance (*sattva*), action (*rajas*), and reaction (*tamas*). (5)

We have the opportunity in our lives to respond or rest in any of these three states: the neutral, clear, calm sattvic place of mind; the fiery outwardly-oriented active rajasic state; and the cool watery inwardly-oriented protective tamasic state. And often we go back and forth between all three. Each is needed. Or, as Dr. Stone wrote, "*Energy in motion anywhere must have this triple action in order to function.*" (6)

THE CURRENTS IN MOVEMENT

CURRENT:	ASSOCIATED GUNA:	MOVEMENT IN SPACE:	CAN BE USED TO BALANCE:
Transverse or East-West current	*Sattva*	side to side	Vata, air Breathing
Spiral or Umbilicus current	*Rajas*	forward and backward	Pitta, fire Tonify digestive fire
Long Line currents	*Tamas*	up and down	Kapha, water Emotional patterns (Air & ether long lines can help balance Vata) (Fire long line can be used to clear Pitta)

The following images are another way to understand how the gunas can express in terms of their qualities of movement:

Sattva
light, delicate, clear, graceful
you move like a pure almost still pond basking in the sunlight
your waters swaying quietly in rhythm with a nearly
imperceptible breeze

Rajas
dynamic, insistent, dashing, passionate
you move like a stallion around a mare in heat
forward and back, forward and back, yearning

Tamas
heavy-footed, bulky, strong, unyielding
you move like a 600 year old oak in winter
its sap moving up and down its trunk in an infinitely
slow dance of nurturance

Randolph Stone described tamas in the following way: *"Tamas is the attractive power of the negative pole of energy emanation, the moon-type energy of cooling, green rays— the feminine precipitating, centralizing, toning and quieting principle, the nest-building instinct in all living things, which becomes resistant to change."* (7)

The gunas manifest in all of life, including Dr. Stone's "Wireless Energy Currents." The transverse current, also known as the east-west current, is an expression of sattva. Dr. James Said, DC, ND, RPP has described it well: "The transverse current emanates from the caduceus pattern of the chakras, going out through the perineum as two sideways spinning spirals, one spinning to the right, the other to the left. These two gyrating currents spiral down around the body and then back up to return to the caduceus through the top of the head." (See illustration, The Transverse Current.) If you imagine yourself standing in a giant double toy "Slinky" made of light in a roughly basket-like shape, you have a rough approximation of the transverse current's pulsation.

The transverse current is a neutral airy energy which helps clear and calm our core as well as support our parasympathetic nervous system. Dr. Said has described it as an information-gathering system, keeping watch over our energy field and taking in information as needed from our external environment. Its sattvic neutral quality supports peace of mind and meditation. It affects all organs and all five oval fields of the body, allowing us to adjust in an integrated and coherent manner with our full organism. Energetically, Dr. Damon Fazio, ND, RPP, has pointed out the similarity between the path of the transverse current and the shape of the rib cage protecting the lungs, thereby relating this current to the intake of air and prana. (8)

Transverse or East-West Current

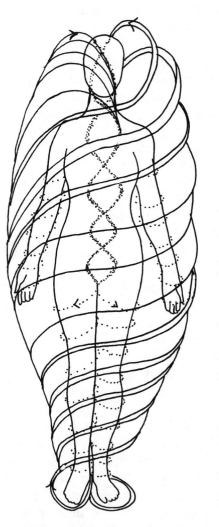

Based in part on ideas in an illustration by Mark Allison, in *Esoteric Anatomy* by Bruce Burger, p. 18, with appreciation.

In my experience as a Polarity Therapist and Ayurvedic nutritionist, it appears that working with the transverse current positively affects the Ayurvedic dosha known as Vata. Supporting the free flow of energy in this current helps both calm Vata and clear obstructions in its flow. This current reveals itself in our side-to-side movements. (9)

The Spiral or Umbilicus Current

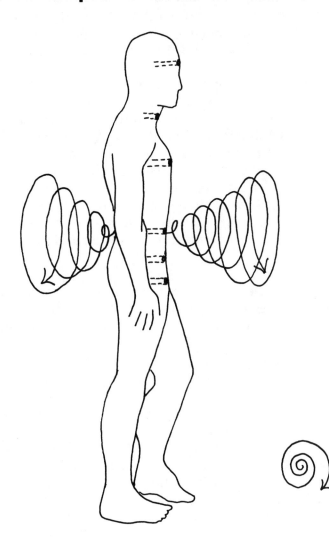

The spiral current, also known as the umbilical current, is rajasic in impulse. It is the current that motivates the body to move. It arises out of the third chakra, spiraling out from the navel and back (upper lumbar, between L-2 and L-3) simultaneously in two right-rotating spirals, as Said has described. The spiral current pulses outward away from our bodies both forward and back with a fiery warming energy (see illustration, The Spiral Current). It enlivens our digestive system and is a source of positive, assertive expansive energy. It is an expression of rajas, and supports the sympathetic nervous system in its function. (10)

Working with the spiral current enhances Pitta dosha, enabling it to effectively express in a calm clear way. When balanced, the spiral current can warm us up without burning us up. Obstructions in the flow of the spiral current can negatively impact Pitta, allowing this dosha to accumulate to an excess, as congested inflammation, or to stagnate, as poor digestion, to name a couple of specific examples. Hence, a free flow of energy through the spiral current also helps Pitta and a healthy digestive fire. The spiral current relates to movements forward and backward, on all levels. (11)

The long line currents are inherently tamasic; they hold our stored memories. (Together all three currents hold our history of unresolved charges.) The long lines arise individually from each of the five lower chakras, creating long lines of energy, which flow upward and downward from top to bottom along our bodies, relating to each of the five elements through these chakras, arising from them and returning to them. (See illustration, The Long Lines Current) In describing the long lines emerging from the chakras, Polarity Therapist Lee has likened their motion to that of a spinning Chinese firecracker. Imagine a watery wheel spinning clockwise in space, sending off spray or "sparks". This spray is the long lines, propelled about the body and back to the chakras, within our core. (12)

The Long Lines Current—Front

Ether chakra spins out ether long lines

The long line currents collectively support the overall well being of our physical bodies, our central nervous system, and our craniosacral rhythms. James Said has said that they enable information to be carried between the five oval fields of the body (see chapter 1). He has also described how the long lines set up the physiology of the body to act based on our conscious and subconscious desires. This system has a relationship with what psychoneuroimmunologist Candace Pert calls "molecules of emotion". The long lines set up a field moving upward and downward, with information coming in through the senses, and our responses going out as motor impulses. (13)

The Long Lines Current—Back

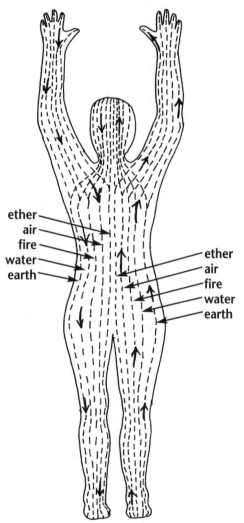

Based on Stone, *Polarity Therapy, Vol. II,* p. 102

The long lines have a watery, cooling, fluid, tamasic energy as a whole. In another way of looking at this, Franklyn Sills, in *The Polarity Process* has pointed out that, "Dr. Stone said that the Long Line Currents carry the energies of the mind into the body and hence govern the functioning of the five senses." (14)

The long lines are an excellent way to access beliefs, feelings, and Kapha dosha, positively affecting healing. Since each of the long lines relates to an element through the chakras, it is possible to use air and ether long lines to help clear Vata blockages, and the fire long line to support Pitta. There is a Polarity Toe Balance process presented later in this chapter as a way you can work with the long line currents for yourself. The long line currents reveal themselves in movements that flow top to bottom, up and down. (15)

Together, the three currents create our place in spatial reality, each delineating one of the three dimensions: the transverse current, in side to side motion; the spiral current, in front and backward motion; and the long lines in their movement upward and downward. (16)

CORE AND PERIPHERY:

Each of the three currents arises from the core, our internal chakra system, and flows out to the periphery and back. Some of us tend to hold more of our energy in the core, while others extend a larger percentage of this energy to the periphery of the current, the outer edges of our fields. How this energy tends to run and accumulate in each of us can have a strong effect on how we feel. What is important to understand here is that each current flows outward and returns back inward. The combination of the three currents create the whole. (17) For more about working with your core and periphery, see chapter 8.

POLARITY: LOCATING OUR ENERGY TWISTS AND TURNS

This next process is based on the assumption that sometimes our unconscious minds know more about what's going on in our physical and energetic bodies than we might realize. You'll need a pen or pencil and some paper for this one.

First draw three pictures of your body, as tiny or large as you like. Once you've done these three quick sketches, draw each of the three energy currents, one for each drawing of your body. If you need help remembering what the energy currents look like, you can refer back to the illustrations here in this chapter. For example, around your first picture of your body, draw a rough approximation of the east-west current. Around the second, you draw the spiral current, around the third, the long lines. Don't worry too much about perfect accuracy or how well you can or can't draw, just have fun and draw them as you like, your version of what you think they are like.

When you feel complete to your satisfaction (or exasperation?), look at your pictures. Are there any breaks in your lines? Where are they? Is one side or part of your body more emphasized than another? Again, not to worry if it is. This is information, and often useful input. For example, did you draw the long lines bigger on your right side than on your left? Check to see if the left leg is shorter than the right. Often times it will be in this situation, because as Dr. Stone pointed out, a constriction in the long lines on one side can show up as a contraction in the muscles (usually in the pelvis) on the same side. Too wild? Try another one: is your transverse current drawn in (literally) around your chest and expanded around your hips? See whether your chest and shoulders are contracted and weight has settled into your hips. How about a break in the long lines? This often can indicate a place that is a bit neglected, or cut off from the flow, so to speak.

Once you have received this information from your hand and body, you can play with it as you like. You can move with that area, or breathe into it, talk with it, sing to it. More information follows on how to work with each of the three currents.

THREE CURRENT CHI GUNG:

Three Current Chi Gung is a good way to begin to explore the currents. This can be done pretty much anywhere with an open mind and comfortable clothing. With your hands about an inch or so from your body, you will be tracing your own energy currents.

TRANSVERSE CURRENT:

For the transverse current, start with your hands with palms facing your forehead (see illustration, Transverse Current Chi Gung). Gently, with your hands close to your body, begin to move them slowly down the front of your body, crisscrossing your hands across your midline, as if you were tracing the pathways of ida and pingala as they nourish the chakras. Let your hands move like two snakes in their side-to-side crisscross motion. Breathe quietly and easily as you move. (18)

Transverse Current Chi Gung

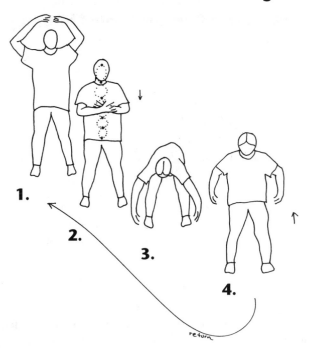

When you have encompassed the whole caduceus, your central channel, as your hands move below your hips and perineum, let your hands make their way all the way to your feet. As you get to your feet, let your hands move to the sides of the feet and begin to gather the energy in and up in a side-to-side motion, all the way back up your body. When your hands find themselves hovering above your head, gently bat the energy toward the crown of your head, as if you were sending energy into a basket. Notice how you feel. You may find your whole body wanting to move from side-to-side, that's fine. Do this slow side-to-side movement as many times as you like, at least two or three times to start. I like to finish with one hand on the center of my chest and the other on my back near my kidneys. You can finish by resting your hands on your body wherever it feels appropriate to you, with your knees slightly relaxed. This particular process can be quite relaxing and calming. If you like, you can combine this movement with a mantra such as RAM, chanted inwardly or out loud.

Transverse Current Chair Chi Gung

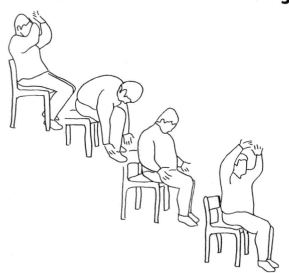

If your back or knees aren't ready yet to stretch down in the forward movement toward your feet, you can try the same process sitting in a chair, going over as far as feels comfortable for you. (See illustration, Transverse Current Chair Chi Gung.) The point is to make contact with your own transverse current and its side-to-side motion. Do not be too concerned about what you can feel or not as you first begin to do this; simply let yourself be moved by the energy of the current.

Spiral Current Chi Gung

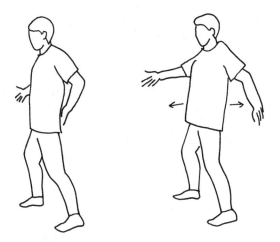

SPIRAL CURRENT:

For the spiral current, stand with your feet about shoulder-width apart, knees relaxed. Place your right hand about an inch or so away from your navel, palm facing in. Rest your left hand on your back at your waist, palm facing in toward your right hand. Slowly begin to move your right hand forward and backward, letting your left hand rest where it is. Breath deeply. After a few moments, you can put your right foot forward and let your body rock slowly backward and forward between your two feet. As you do this, (I swear it's easier to do than to read) slowly let your right hand expand its movement into a larger and larger clockwise spiral (see illustration, Spiral Current Chi Gung). If you are feeling energetic, you might want to see what it feels like to continue this spiraling hand movement while you walk slowly forward and backward, or let both hands move, the one in front, the other in back. You can say "HA!" to increase energy. Or for a more calming effect, use a silent or vocalized SHRIM as you move.

VARIATIONS: If you're practicing from a chair or wheelchair, you can work with the same movement while seated. You can also experiment with bringing your chest forward and back (or thinking your chest forward and back) to get a sense of what it feels like to expand into the spiral current (forward) and to retract back into it (backward).

For a more energetic experience, seated or standing, try quietly saying "HA" with every breath and movement. Or try hollering "HA" at the top of your lungs!

Spiral Current Chair Chi Gung

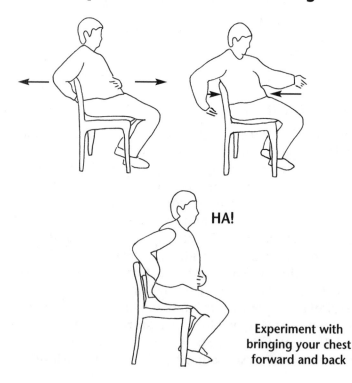

HA!

Experiment with
bringing your chest
forward and back

LONG LINES:

Working with the long lines is initially a little more complicated to learn, yet ultimately quite fun. At first these moves may feel like trying to do the combined set of goofy movements of patting one's head while doing a circular motion with the other hand on the belly. That is, in Long Lines Current Chi Gung, each hand is moving independently up and down. It gets easier rapidly as you do it a few times.

Long Lines Current Chi Gung

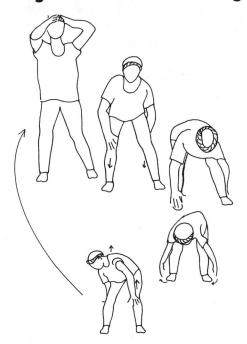

You begin with your hands close to the top of your head. Your right palm is just above your right eye and your left palm faces the back of the left side of your head (see illustration, Long Lines Current Chi Gung). Both hands begin to slowly move down your body, the right hand moving down the front of the RIGHT side of your body while your left hand simultaneously moves down the LEFT side of your back. When you get down to your feet, bending your knees a bit if you need to, your hands simultaneously rotate around each foot in a clockwise direction, so that the right hand moves from facing the right toes to facing the right heel, while the left hand moves around from facing the left heel to facing the left toes. You then bring your hands UP your body, the right hand now coming up the right side in the back, while the left hand is moving up the front of your body on the left side. Your hands never cross over one another; the right hand stays on the right side of the body, the left hand on the left side. When your hands reach your head again, they continue on over close to the head, the right heading toward the front again, the left to the back. This is one circuit. You can try 3 or 4 times at whatever pace feels comfortable to you. OM is beneficial to chant with this movement, if you like, aloud or inside.

Long Lines Current Chair Chi Gung

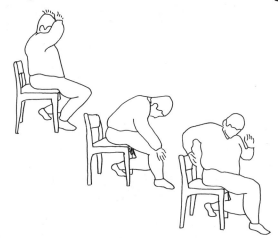

The same process can be done from a chair, if you need to do it this way. The model for Long Lines Current Chair Chi Gung, is Polarity Therapist Louise Henry, a disability counselor who has also worked with a fused hip since childhood. She and I wanted to demonstrate in this sequence that the priority here is to come in contact with the currents however you can, rather than to try to maintain some perfect externalized form. To be able to reach as much of the long line current as she can, Henry moves her left leg backward. You might do it differently. The point of this process is to begin to contact the energy, however that works for you.

CONTINUING EXPLORATION OF THE CURRENTS:

The following simple stretches can help you get more acquainted with the directional movements associated with the currents. Again, you're in comfortable clothing, loose or stretchy, in a comfortable space. This whole series of stretches takes about ten minutes to do. It is a good preliminary for either of the routines that follow, the first to relax and focus, the second to energize.

Opening Stretches

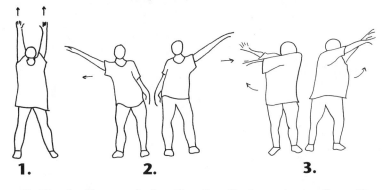

1.   **2.**   **3.**

1) Physically: reach for the sky, first one arm, then the other, alternating the stretch in each arm, 6-12 times. Then massage your head and neck.

Energetically: you are following the long line currents, up and down as you move your arms.

2) Physically: with feet shoulder-width apart and planted firmly on the ground, knees relaxed and a little bent, reach out to the side, first in one direction, then the other. Stretch first your right arm as far as you can to your right, then your left arm to your left, stretching and reaching

Energetically: you are connecting with the side-to-side movement of the transverse current

3) Physically: feet still shoulder-width apart, swing your arms together from one side to the other and back, 6-12 times. Relax and breathe as you do.

Energetically: you are following the transverse current in its side-to-side movements again.

Opening Stretches

4.

5.

6.

4) Physically: stand relaxed with your feet about 6″ apart. Put one foot forward, leaving the other foot with the heel flat on the ground (that's where the stretch is, in your calf). Hold 15 seconds or as long as it is comfortable, alternate with your other foot forward. This can also be done up against the wall. (Note: This stretch is a slight variation on one from Bob Anderson's excellent book, *Stretching*. The next stretch is also in his book. (19)

Energetically: you can imagine moving with the spiral current, as you move forward, then back. From standing, gather the energy inward and downward with your hands as you sit down for the next stretch.

5) Physically: come to sitting on the ground, with the soles of your feet pressed together. Lightly grasp your feet with your hands and gently bend forward with a straight back from your hips. The stretch is in your groin and inner thighs. Look a little in front of you as you relax and breathe. Hold 15-20 seconds, relax, repeat.

Energetically: imagine the spiral current radiating out from your umbilicus (navel) as you bend forward. You can try expanding into the spiral current as you inhale, and relax with the exhale. This can be quite warming.

6) Physically: you will be easing into Dr. Stone's (famous) Squat: with feet even, parallel with each other about 18" apart, slowly work yourself toward the ground by leaning forward or rocking up and down. If you can, relax yourself into a squat with both feet flat on the floor. Reach your hands out for balance at first, not resting on the floor. If this is too hard, let yourself grab a stable chair or the legs of a desk for support as you adjust yourself to squatting. Or you can lean your back lightly against a wall. (20) If a friend is there, try holding hands as you each face one another squatting: much easier, yes? (See illustration, Variations on Squats, A)

Some people find a wide stance is easier to get into, as in position B. Others prefer wrapping their arms around their legs, as in position C. Some squatting positions encourage introspection, like positions D and E. In D, you hold your head between your hands, which can feel remarkably comforting. In E, the area along the eye socket can be worked to release tension and toxins, or simply held, to gather your focus inside.

Energetically: there are many areas you can become aware of, as you stretch in a squat. You can play with rocking front to back, with your arms around your legs with the spiral current. Or you can move side-to-side, swaying a bit with the transverse current.

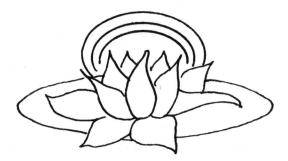

Variations on Squats

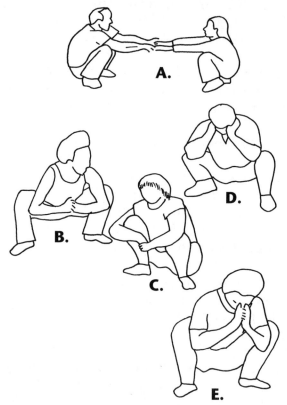

The key to the squat is gentle motion; it is harder to do the more stationary you are. Relax; let yourself discover which parts of you move easily and which don't. If you can't get all the way down, know you're in good company! Stretch into it as much as you comfortable can. In a number of weeks, you may surprise yourself with your agility.

EVOLUTION AND INVOLUTION

Dr. Stone observed two other basic patterns of posture and movement, which are easy to incorporate as simple stretches. He called them evolutionary and involutionary.

Evolution & Involution

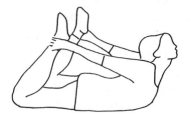

Evolutionary Stretch
–return to formless spirit–

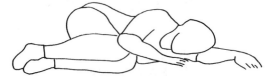

Involutionary Stretch
–spirit into form–

In evolutionary postures, like the back bend or any other backward stretch, we are releasing ourselves, opining to the new, moving back into a deeper alignment with formless spirit, from the Polarity perspective. (21) This same backward stretch is used by some chiropractors to invite the gel around the discs of our spines to rearrange into more effective cushioning patterns for our discs. The evolutionary stretch pictured here is the yogic Bow, traditionally called Dhanurahsana.

An easy example of an involutionary pattern is letting yourself curl up comfortably in a little ball. This mimics the posture we had prenatally in our mothers' wombs. It is involutionary in that we are coming into form, moving more deeply into the realities of the physical world.

SynergyDance uses this fetal position for vital "resourcing", letting your energy and resources flow back in and around you. Usually this fetal position is done lying on ones' left side with a pillow under the head, or using one's arm as a pillow. It is a good way to complete your series of stretches. Take a few minutes to breath deeply, let yourself rest in this position for three minutes at least. Dr. Stone maintained that taking this fetal position for just a few minutes every day allows all three currents to flow freely and promotes good health. Our aim is to let all three currents cooperate. Balance comes when all three currents are flowing freely; no one current dominates. (22)

The sun salute, the traditional series of yoga asanas from India, is another excellent example of movements which incorporate both involutionary and evolutionary patterns. (23)

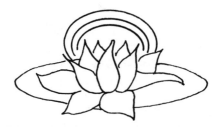

POLARITY YOGA STRETCHES:

Dr. Stone devoted a substantial part of his self-care book, *Health Building: The Conscious Art of Living Well* to yoga stretches he had developed specifically to free up energy, which he called "health postures". These original stretches tone both your currents and your muscles. Two sequences, both of which include the preceding warm-up moves, are given here. One is to relax and focus, the other to energize.

Each generation is unique in its perspectives and needs. What I have noticed in my practice in the last few years is that younger people born in the 1970's and 19809's have a deep transformative potential, as well as a remarkable ability to trap tension. I have been surprised to see so much tension in people so young. The relaxing sequence that follows would be useful for any age, if you are dealing with tension or over-stimulation of the nervous system.

Stone emphasized that to get the fullest benefit from the postures, you need to stay present with the stretches and your breath. The purpose is to activate and free up the flow of the currents, rather than simply to develop muscle or flexibility, although these results do follow with practice. *"It is a path of life rather than of force; of rest rather than of conquest....It is like turning on a switch and allowing the currents to do the work..."* (24)

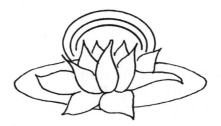

A POLARITY YOGA ROUTINE TO RELAX AND FOCUS:

Do the first five opening stretches (pp. 71 & 72) to limber up, with a bit of a shift as you stretch: imagine that you are a five-pointed star, with your head, hands and feet the five points. As you stretch up and out, let all the points of your star stretch. When you do the second stretch, with each arm reaching to the side, notice the diagonal stretch happening between your shoulder and the opposite hip. Imagine you are activating a smaller five-pointed star with its points being your head, shoulders and hips.

In doing the last couple of preliminary stretches, let yourself notice what it is like to become a five-pointed star with spirals emerging from your belly and back. See what happens to the spirals as you lean forward and back. Then, from the fifth stretch sitting on the floor, let yourself move into the following gentle stretch from Dr. Stone (25):

Polarity Yoga to Relax & Focus

1. Motor Balance Posture

2. The Cobra

1) Physically: sitting on the floor with your knees up, legs together, and feet flat on the floor, let your spine relax as you sit. Your fingers are interlaced behind your neck as you breathe naturally. Let your knees relax so that they can easily support your elbows.

Energetically: notice your curved-inward posture, like the fetal position earlier. Let yourself imagine you are coming fully into form (involutionary).

2) Physically: we will be doing the Cobra. Using your back and abdominal muscles, arch backward. Keep your neck and arms relaxed. To encourage extra relaxation in your neck and head, be sure and start with your head resting on its side, turning to the front as you inhale into the stretch. Exhale back to the floor, face looking to the opposite side. (26)

Energetically: this offers a counter-pose to the preceding stretch, and invites us to move into the new (evolutionary).

3) Physically: stay on your tummy with your head resting on your arms. You will be doing a Scissors Kick with your legs. Start with your legs extended outward, then let your legs crisscross inward, out and in, out and in. I think of this as the windshield-wiper move. Repeated for a couple of minutes to up to ten minutes, Stone used this exercise to clear the sinuses and relieve head congestion. (27)

Energetically: there are a number of fun things to explore here. You can tune in on the long lines, and notice what happens as your legs crisscross. Or you can see what happens to your five-pointed star as you move in this way. You can also imagine the chakras radiating up your spine and the flow of the transverse current as it flows out of the perineum and moves around and up your body, re-entering at the crown of your head. (28)

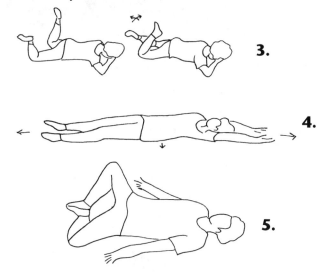

4) Physically: roll over on to your back. Stretch your arms high above your head, resting them on the floor. As you inhale, press your back flat against the floor at the small of your back, pointing your toes and reaching with your arms as you do, as if you were trying to get as long and flat as you possibly can. Exhale as your relax and let go of the stretch. Do 3-6 times.

Energetically: imagine your five-pointed star is lengthening and flattening as you do this one.

5) Physically: still lying on your back, inhale as you bring the soles of your feet together and drop your knees toward the floor. Relax, hold the stretch for 40-60 seconds or as long as comfortable. Let your groin and perineal muscles relax.

Energetically: imagine the long lines running down your arms and legs and returning upward.

Polarity Yoga to Relax & Focus

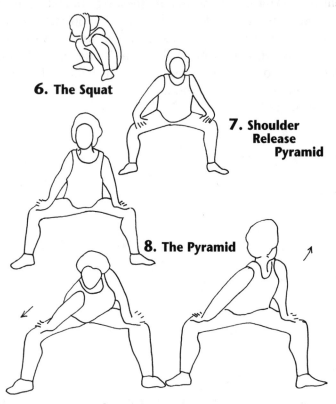

6. The Squat

7. Shoulder Release Pyramid

8. The Pyramid

9. Twisting Pyramid

6) Physically: gently roll to one side, and ease yourself in-to a squat. Your aim, over time, is to get your feet flat on the floor. Let your arms extend out in front of you for balance, or you can use any of the aids mentioned earlier: leaning your back against a wall, holding on to furniture, or balancing with a friend. Rock back and forth, side to side, in slow easy circles.

Energetically: focus on the sensations in your shoulders, back and ankles (Stone's "airy triad") as you stretch and sway.

7) Physically: coming to standing, plant your feet wide apart, solid on the ground. Rest your hands facing forward on your knees and let your neck and back relax. You are supporting your spine and head with your arms and legs. Dr. Stone used this posture to relax the hips, back, shoulders, and neck, often stressed spots in our world. He also recommended this posture for headache prevention. (29)

Energetically: return to the image of yourself as a five-pointed star. As your arms resting on your legs support your back completely, let these four points of your star support your center.

8) Physically: staying in the same basic posture, slide your hands parallel with your legs, still resting on the knees. Sway from side-to-side, especially letting the SHOULDERS relax. (30)

Energetically: shift your focus back to the chakras and the energy along your spine, the transverse current encircling you as you sway.

9) Physically: you will be moving from this same position into a posture known as the Twisting Pyramid. Go slowly. Rotate your right shoulder forward and down, simultaneously looking over the shoulder at your right foot. With your right shoulder still forward and down, look up and over your left shoulder. Let your spine relax as you make these moves; it is supported. Repeat on the other side, alternating 2-6 times. (31)

Energetically: experience your five-pointed star as you move.

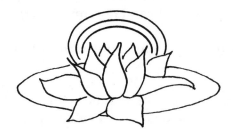

Polarity Yoga to Relax & Focus

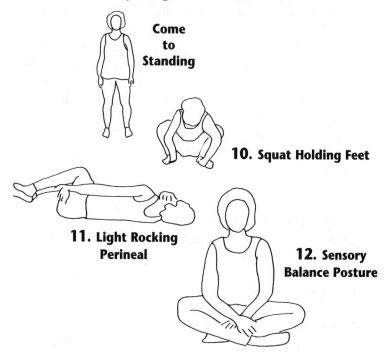

Come to Standing

10. Squat Holding Feet

11. Light Rocking Perineal

12. Sensory Balance Posture

10) Physically: return to standing and ease yourself back into a squat, and if you can, grasp the insides of your feet with your hands. If you can't, let yourself relax as much into the posture as you can, rocking and breathing.

Energetically: ask yourself, what circuits are being completed here?

11) Physically: lie on your right side, with your right arm resting on your jaw or the back of your head, whichever is more comfortable. Left hand rests on the perineum. Breathe and relax.

Energetically: relax and notice whatever sensations come to you.

12) Closing: sit on the ground with your legs crossed, right hand over left, relax and breathe. (32)

A Note: as you move, many sensations and observations may come to you, including possible understandings about the currents and how they operate. This is the excitement of this kind of movement. The questions and guidance offered here are simply ways to get you exploring. You may notice other information than that shared here, which is great. And if you don't happen to notice something mentioned here, not to worry. We're each different, with different experiences. Explore as much as you like.

---

*CAUTION symbol:
Our bodies have histories. Some of us have been injured, or have inherited congenital challenges. Some exercises need to be approached with caution. I've used the same symbol that Chitty & Muller have in their excellent Polarity Yoga book, *Energy Exercises*, to alert you that certain exercises need to be done with caution and care, or avoided entirely. As they have said, "LISTEN TO YOUR BODY FIRST."

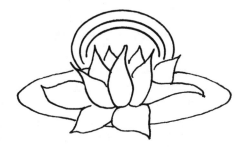

AN ENERGIZING POLARITY YOGA ROUTINE:

Dr. Stone delighted in getting energy flowing through the body with vigorous movements. Many of his most revitalizing postures work with the spiral current and the syllable "HA!" These movements and sounds work with energy much as practitioners of karate work with the hara center and chi.

A HA! story: it may be a little out-moded here in 21st century America, and yet its intent is to convey the energy of "HA!" As you may recall, the spiral current is associated with rajas and creative, outgoing, masculine energy, and HA! stimulates this energy positively. If there's anyone out there who remembers growing up on a farm or visiting one, you may recall what roosters are like. For readers unfamiliar with roosters' behavior, they like to sneak up and ambush the unaware. I have a friend with a small barnyard scene who uses HA! to defend herself. Inevitably, in the course of feeding the animals and gathering the eggs, she faces the free-roaming rooster. She has discovered a well-placed HA!, shouted emphatically from the belly straight at the rooster, stops it dead in its tracks, no matter how vigorous its approach. This is the kind of wild energy you are welcome to bring to the following routine, or to generate with its movements. You may not need to repel a marauding rooster, yet, you will be ready.

NOTE: It is important to do the opening stretches on pp. 71 & 72 even if you are in good shape, so as to warm up the hamstrings and other muscles involved here. The therapist in training who modeled this sequence, Ronaldo Estevan, RPP candidate and LMT candidate, maintains an active body-building program. Yet, he noticed in doing the opening stretches that they simultaneously relaxed and stretched areas that he didn't always work in his regular exercise program. This program is relatively demanding on the back, knees, and shoulders; be realistic and keep in touch with your own limits.

Polarity Yoga to Energize

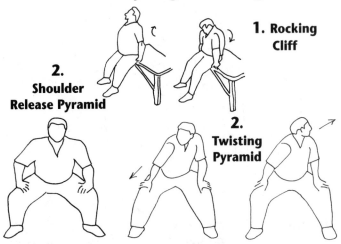

2. Shoulder Release Pyramid

1. Rocking Cliff

2. Twisting Pyramid

1) Physically: this first posture slowly and gently opens the chest and back. It can be done on a tallish stool, massage table or piano bench, or even on the side of a bed. You sit with feet flat on the floor, arms holding the edge of the bench. Let the head relax. Rock yourself back and forth using your arms, chest and back muscles, 6-12 times. This stretch has been called the Rocking Cliff. (33)

Energetically: notice the difference between chest out (evolutionary) and chest pulled in (involutionary).

2) Physically: you will be moving into the Pyramid, presented in the RELAXING routine. With feet positioned wide and firmly apart, rest your hands and fingers forward on your knees. Rotate your right shoulder forward and down, simultaneously twisting your head to gaze over your right shoulder at your right foot. With your right shoulder still forward, look up and over your left shoulder. Let your spine relax as you make these moves; it is supported by your arms and hands. Repeat on the other side, bringing your left shoulder forward and stretching to look at your left foot, then looking up and over your right shoulder. Alternate 2-6 times. This is an effective spinal twist that is good for relieving fatigue.

Energetically: notice where energy gathers for you in this posture.

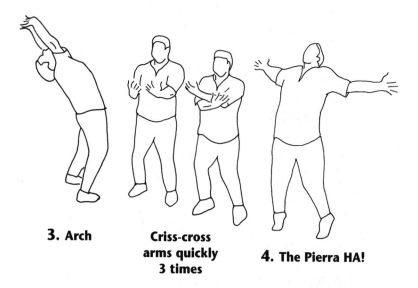

3. Arch   **Criss-cross
arms quickly
3 times**   **4. The Pierra HA!**

3) Physically: stand with feet shoulder-width apart, or a
little wider. Stretch your arms high over your head as you
arch backward. Knees are slightly bent. Breathe deeply. It is
normal for the muscles to tremble some on this one.
   Energetically: notice how the center of your chest and
navel feel. Relax.

4) Physically: this next stretch has been called the
Pierre HA!, after Polarity Therapist and teacher Pierre
Pannetier. It is fun for people of all ages. Stand with your
arms in front of you, palms up, and quickly cross them,
right over left, left over right, etc. three times. Then
throw your arms out to your sides with a loud HA! on exhale. You can get into quite a rhythm of 1-2-3-HA! When
you feel confident of your balance in this movement,
you can try coming up on your toes with the exhaling
HA! (34)
   Energetically: check out how this affects your spiral current and the area around your navel and lumbar spine.

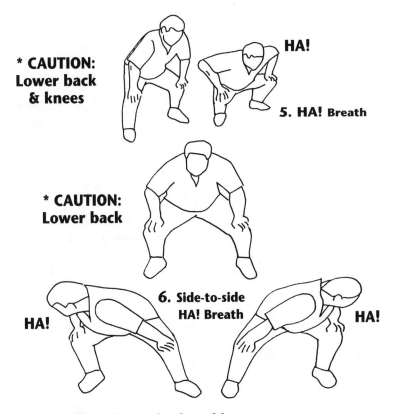

5) * CAUTION: lower back and knees
Physically: position yourself as you would for the
Pyramid, feet wide apart, hands on knees. Inhale, and come
down as low as you can, close to squatting, on the exhale
with a HA! Let your head relax. Inhale again as you come up,
exhale down with a HA! Dr. Stone used this to release tension
in the shoulders and neck, as well as to strengthen digestion
and the kidneys, and move overall sluggishness. (35)
Energetically: notice the long lines and spiral current.

6) * CAUTION: lower back
Physically: coming from the same position, inhale and
then exhale with a HA! as you bend over your right leg.
Alternate sides, inhaling as you rise, exhaling with a HA! as
you bend. This has been called a Side to Side HA stretch. (36)
Energetically: notice the spiral current as you move. Do
you get warmer?

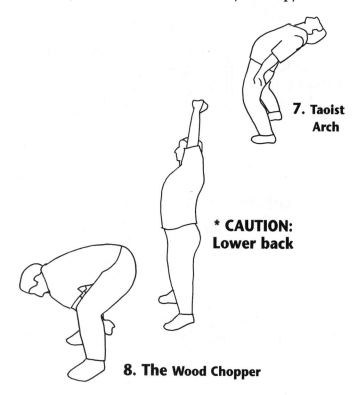

7. Taoist
    Arch

* CAUTION:
Lower back

8. The Wood Chopper

7) Physically: stand up straight, with your arms at your sides. In a relaxing counter-pose to the last couple of stretches, let your body relax backward in a Taoist arch. Feet are about shoulder-width apart. Again, your muscles may tremble some in this position; it's one normal response. (37)
Energetically: notice what it feels like to hold this open posture.

8)*CAUTION: lower back
Physically: stand with your hands clasped over your head, feet shoulder width apart. Inhale, and with a HA! on the exhale, bring your arms vigorously down, as if you were chopping wood. (This exercise is often called the Wood Chopper.) Let the movement come from your pelvis, with your arms following the pelvis. Repeat 3-6 times. (38)
Energetically: notice your relative degree of warmth, before and after this exercise.

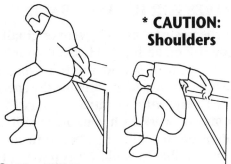

*** CAUTION:
Shoulders**

9. The Cliff Hanger

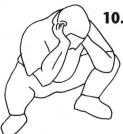

**10. The Youth Posture:
Humming Squat**

9) *CAUTION: shoulders

Physically: feet flat on the ground, rest your weight on y-our hands as they hold on to a low bench or bar behind you (it is also possible to do this with a low massage table). Simply hold the stretch with a relaxed head and neck, without letting your buttocks rest on the ground. Breathe naturally. Known as the Cliff Hanger, Stone used this to tonify the lower back, hips, shoulders, and activate digestion. (39)

Energetically: key in on the relationships between your throat, heart, and belly as you hold the posture.

10) Closing, physically: let yourself relax into a squat, however you can. This particular posture Stone called the Youth Posture for its revitalizing effects. Rest your elbows on your knees and place your little fingers in your ears. With eyes closed, begin to hum, until you find a pitch that feels soothing or enlivening to you. (40)

Energetically: imagine you are giving yourself a Polarity treatment. The focus of your attention is your two little fingers. As you hum, let the energy balance between your hands.

ALTERNATIVES FOR HEALING BACKS:

Several of the postures as they were originally presented can put undue risk on an injured back. If your back falls into this category, you may find the following alternatives offer you the opportunity to experience the energetic aspect of the posture safely, without hurting yourself. No need to be macho or macha; work with your own reality. Once I was limping ignominiously with my bag into an airport far from home, barely able to walk. I was praying to get home with my back in one (movable) piece. The airline attendant behind the counter took in my whole story with one compassionate glance; I hadn't said a word yet. "You know," he said, "a back is like an ankle or anything else. Once you sprain or strain it, it can happen again. You gotta be careful." He was right. Backs need to be rebuilt wisely, like any other part of us.

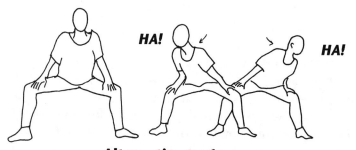

Alternative to 6:
Side-to-side HA! Break

Alternatives for Healing Backs

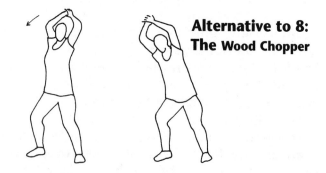

Alternative to 8:
The Wood Chopper

Alternative to 6: take the same position, but bend from the hips, not the back. Keep the back straight as you exhale with a HA!, only going as far down as it feels comfortable for your back.

Alternative to 8: take the same position as in the Wood Chopper, with your arms over your head. Instead of swinging your arms down to the floor, focus your attention in your pelvis. The movement is in the pelvis for this alternative move, not in the back. Inhale with your arms over your head, exhale with a HA!, contracting your pelvis as you do (see illus). Send the HA! out through your belly, keeping your legs loose and relaxed. DON'T bend in the lower back, and only bring your arms over your head as far as is comfortable for your back.

Energetically on Alternative 8: let yourself key in on the evolutionary bend inherent in the starting position and the involutionary posture of the HA! exhale.

These routines are one way to play. To experience the original stretches from Dr. Stone for yourself, see *Health Building*, pp. 130–187. If you find yourself inspired by this yoga and want to explore further, see John Chitty and Mary Louise Muller's excellent book on Polarity movement called *Energy Exercises: Easy Exercises for Health and Vitality*. It offers a wealth of insights about self-care, with series of exercises centered around key body areas, such as neck and shoulder, chest and heart, and so on. There is also an easy-to-use Polarity Yoga videotape created by Anna Chitty, RPP, with an hour of well-designed stretches to warm you up into postures that benefit all three currents and all the elements. (See RESOURCES)

DANCING WITH THE ELEMENTS:

SynergyDancer Charmaine Lee, RPP, was first inspired to explore dance as Polarity Therapy after reading a section in Dr. Stone's *Health Building: "Rhythmic expressions of song and dance, which use all the bodily forces and muscles for expression, free the emotions by naturally liberating the energy blocks, suppressions, frustrations and stagnations. And when mind, body and emotions are used in one effort of rhythmic exercise, it becomes a triune health movement of balance."* (41) Over the past fifteen years, Charmaine has been exploring and teaching how the currents clear with movement, and how the currents create movement in us.

SOME KEY UNDERSTANDINGS ABOUT SYNERGYDANCE INCLUDE:

1) Any movement you make needs to begin from inside, move outward and return. This way you are involving all three principles. For a simple example we've used before: Feel your arm. Move it away from you. Bring it back in close. You've done it: sattva/air principle: inner awareness, rajas/fire principle: outer expansion, tamas/water principle: return.

2) To allow the movement to begin from within, take time to resource. Typically, in an hour and a half SynergyDance class, the first 45 minutes would be spent in inwardly-oriented resourcing. How to resource? See below.

3) Let your shoulders and hips move simultaneously. In any move, let both shoulders and hips move. Based on Dr. Stone's work, Charmaine finds this directly moves blockages in the energy current.

4) The goal is to contact energy instead of muscle. (42)

SYNERGYDANCE RESOURCING: HOW TO

Your aim here is to let the energy build through the physical body and be expressed in authentic movements from your core.

Physically: lie on your back with your knees bent, feet flat on the floor. Make contact with your core by placing your right hand on your sacrum, your left hand on the base of your skull. (Alternatively, you can place your right hand on your pubic bone and your left in the center of your forehead.) Breathe in and out naturally, keying in on the sensations of your body. Using your feet to push off into movement, let your sacrum begin to rock down and up. As your spine moves in a rhythmic way, bring your arms up over your head and down around your body. As your arms come up, your knees head more or less toward the sky. As they come down around your sides, your legs naturally open, the knees moving toward the floor. Lee uses this movement to access the craniosacral rhythms of the body, to establish the fluid core, as she calls it.

Energetically: you are relaxing and keying in to the energy of your body. You are letting yourself access your core and the movement of the long lines before you move out into larger movements.

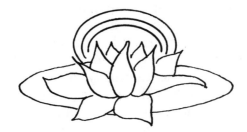

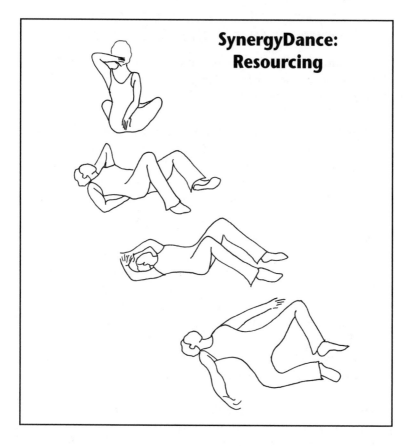

SynergyDance: Resourcing

Resourcing may seem like a subtle movement, and yet it can have profound effects. One colleague of mine, a skilled yoga teacher and bodyworker, told me a story that demonstrates this. A person of enormous energy, she had been practicing yoga for close to thirty years and keeping a full schedule of clients, when her life was disrupted by an auto accident. The whiplash drained her body and mind, an unheard-of experience for my friend. All she could do was lie around. Adapting to her extremely changed circumstances, she decided to work with the energies of the spine and make what micro-movements she could, literally the same sort of rocking pelvic movements described above. After several days of doing little else, she was shocked to experience a surge of energy into her adrenals as she lay watching television, and her old energy entirely returned.

After resourcing, one can begin to contact the elements in the body with larger movements. In one of Lee's workshops that I attended, she put on music to evoke a particular element such as fire. She then invited participants to begin to move each of the three parts of the body related to fire: the head, the belly (solar plexus), and thighs (for more information about these correspondences, see table below).

MOVEMENT, THE BODY, AND THE ELEMENTS: TRIAD WORK

Element:	Body Area:	Astrological Sign:
Air	shoulders kidneys (lower back) ankles	Gemini Libra Aquarius
Fire	head, especially the eyes solar plexus thighs	Aries Leo Sagittarius
Water	breast, chest pelvis, gonads feet	Cancer Scorpio Pisces
Earth	neck lower abdomen knees	Taurus Virgo Capricorn

(45)

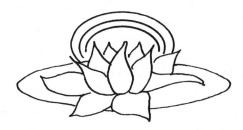

At home, you can do the same thing. On a comfortable warm rug, give yourself time to resource as described. When you feel centered and ready to dance from this space, you might begin by playing some favorite fiery music. Begin to move your head in rhythm with your inner core. Let the movement extend down into your solar plexus, so that your head and belly are moving together. Finally invite your thighs to join the dance, creating a personal dance of fire. Moving backward and forward also puts you in touch with the spiral current, enhancing your connection with your more fiery energies. Notice how your hips and shoulders automatically begin to move as the rest of you does. This kind of fire triad workout both expresses fire and supports a healthy build up of digestive fire.

African dance offers many vibrant examples of how to do such "triad work" in a creative way. Working on your own, you can put on favorite music, and do a fluid "water" dance, moving especially with your chest, your pelvis and your feet. Or a slow and ponderous "earth" dance, focusing on your neck, belly (bowels) and knees. A light and expansive "air" dance would center its movement in your shoulders, back and waist (the kidney/adrenal area) and ankles. (43) Certified SynergyDance teacher Laurie Forbes, RPP, LMT, has modeled some possible elemental dances in the illustrations that follow. (44)

As you play with the dance moves, you may find yourself yearning for more guidance or instruction. There is a SynergyDance video available, as well as trainings, listed in the RESOURCES section which follows.

AIR

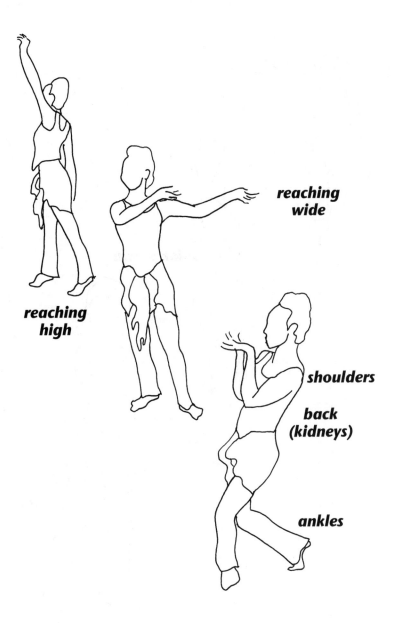

reaching
wide

reaching
high

shoulders

back
(kidneys)

ankles

FIRE

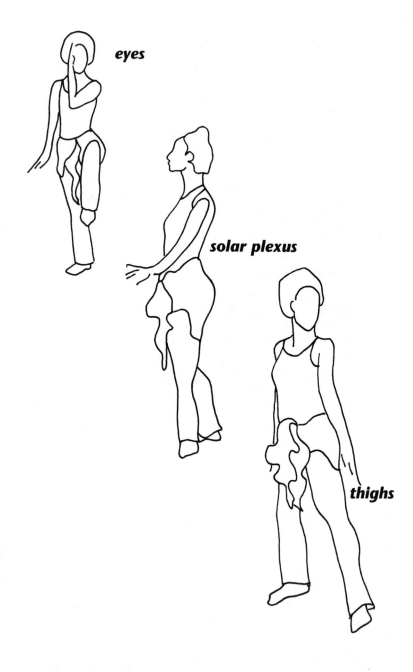

eyes

solar plexus

thighs

WATER

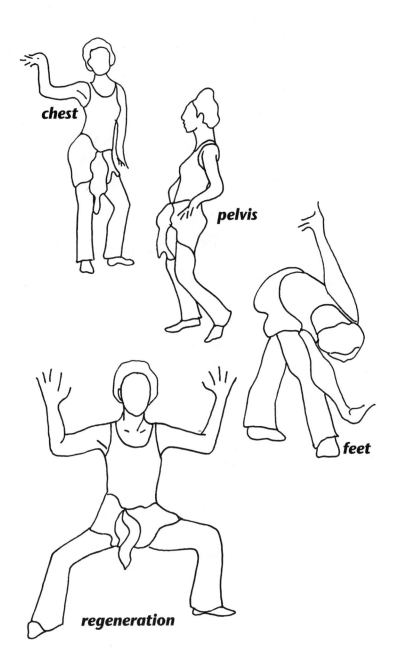

EARTH

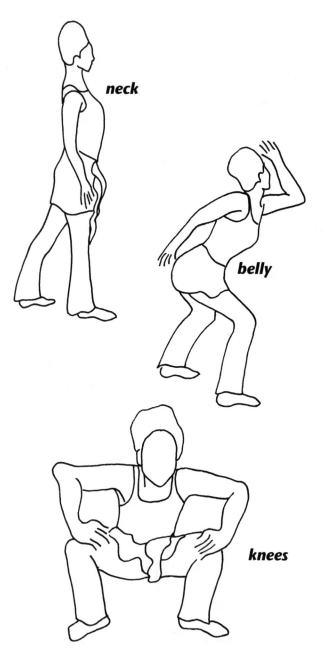

TOE BALANCE:

This final process is deceptively simple, and at first you may think nothing is "happening", so to speak. Yet to put it into context, Dr. Stone valued the information offered in the toes so much that he spent pages describing it. Stone's toe balance is a basic and yet profound technique appreciated by many Polarity Therapy practitioners, and one you can do relatively easily on yourself. (46)

The Hands, the Feet, & the Elements

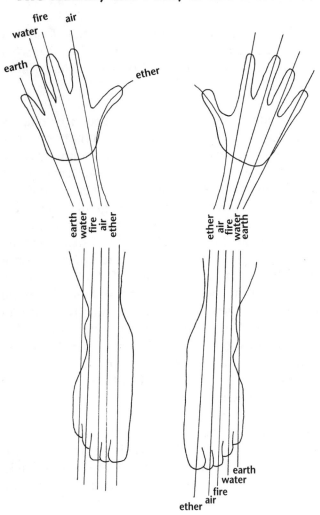

The long line currents of the body wrap along each toe, as well as each finger. Working with the toes can help free up and rebalance congested energies in the long lines. This can also help work with feelings, as the watery long lines have a strong connection with emotion. Working with the feet in general helps ground energy if you are feeling spacey or ungrounded. Working with the toes specifically helps rebalance the relationship of the elements within the body, as each toe through its long line current relates to one of the five elements and the first five chakras. (See illustration, The Hands, the Feet, and the Elements.)

"The fingers and toes become end poles of these over-all currents of sensation and action in the body, directly connected to the center of the Vitality within, to influence it by Polarity balancing." (47)

Seating yourself comfortably on a couch or chair with good back support, bring your legs up so that your toes are in reach of your hands. Wrap your arms around the outside of your legs as you reach for your toes. Your feet can be bare or in socks, whatever feels most comfortable to you.

With your thumbs and forefingers, gently massage your toes for a minute or so, greeting them and letting them know you're about to do a toe balance. Then when you're ready to begin, specifically massage the littlest toe on each foot, using your left hand on your left foot and your right hand on your right foot. Massage these toes for a moment as energetically or gently as suits you, then relax into holding the toes at their bases, between your fingers. It will probably feel most comfortable to have your thumb on the top surface of the foot, your forefinger underneath. As you begin to hold the toes, invite the feet to be a part of balancing the earth element inside.

You may feel nothing as you patiently hold these two little toes or you may feel a lot. Either is normal. After you've held them for what seems like an eon, or possibly the blink of an eye, you may start feeling a pulse in one or both toes.

This is what is known as a "therapeutic pulse", familiar to body workers. When the pulse has arisen in both toes, and both toes' pulses are beating in rhythm, it's time to move on to the next pair of toes. If you feel nothing at all even with patient waiting, don't be daunted. This is not unusual. Often one will grip the toes harder than is needed, especially in our zeal to feel SOMETHING. If you lighten up your pressure, oftentimes a pulse will come forward with this lighter "sattvic" touch. If circulation to the feet is sluggish or this particular element is unused to such attention, your toes may feel almost asleep, like a bear in hibernation. Again, this is not unusual. You can hold the toes as long as you feel able, then move on to the next set of toes, the water toes. Again, ask these toes if they'd like to be a part of balancing the water element in the body, and proceed as before. Some pairs of toes may balance faster than others, this is normal, and offers you information about the balance of elements within your body. When you've gone through each pair of toes all the way to the "ether" (big) toes, you can thank your feet for their participation. You can close with the following gentle hold if you like:

Toe Balance

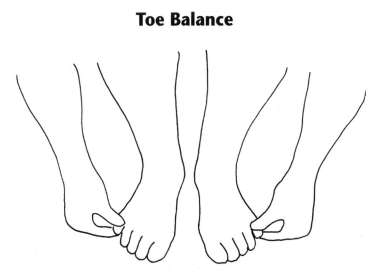

Balancing the Earth Toes

With each thumb resting on the top surface of the foot, place each finger in alignment with its respective toe by resting your finger tips on the bottom base of the toes. You may feel all the toe pulses beating in unison, which is a nice feeling. Close, and relax.

Variation: Baby-Style Toe Balance: You can use this same closing position described above as a starting position for "Baby-Style Toe Balance". Lying on your back on a comfortable warm well-padded surface, bring your feet up as if you were about to play with your toes, which you are. Reaching with your arms INSIDE (medial to) your legs, play with making this same toe hold, each finger in contact with a toe. If you are missing one or more toes, you may still feel the energy there at its base.

You can go on to do the toe balance as described above, letting each element come into balance as it is ready.

FELDENKRAIS MOVEMENT:

In my own adventures with movement and stiffness, I have deeply appreciated the work of Moshe Feldenkrais, who created an independent school of movement unconnected to yoga, Ayurveda, or Polarity per se. As a physicist who began to explore the subtler dimensions of movement when his own knees gave out on him, Feldenkrais' focus was to create pain-free options in movement. This approach offers an accepting, non-judgmental way to accept who we are, and where we can and can't move. His focus was to expand individuals' options, allowing more than one way to get from the chair to the floor and back, for example. Or from lying in bed to standing on both feet. The Feldenkrais method invites us to use more and different muscles, opening to more of who we are. Often we keep moving in one habitual way, not realizing that other movements are available to us, often with much less pain. Feldenkrais can lead us to explore new territories within our own bodies. It can be a valuable adjunct to energy healing, especially if you are working with injuries or aging. (See Alon, RESOURCES)

FACE DANCING

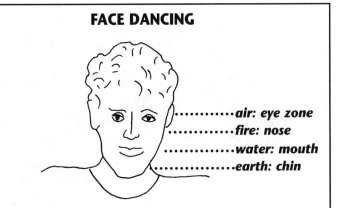

............air: eye zone
............fire: nose
............water: mouth
............earth: chin

Elemental Zones of the Face

Some of us may not want to move our bodies, and yet we may be quite willing to open—our mouths, for example! Face dancing is a goofy activity with unproven clinical possibilities. It is predicated on the hypothesis that having fun could be healing. Face dancing is most fun when done with others, though in a pinch, a mirror will do as witness.

Dr. Stone described four elemental zones in the face; see above. (48) To face dance (I've got to confess, this is my idea, not Dr. Stone's): try to move just one zone at a time, putting as much energy into it as you like. You can move your eyes (air), then your nose (fire), your mouth (water), and your chin (earth).

If you want to explore further, try different movements in each area: how easy is it to move that mouth side to side? Or that nose up and down? How mobile is that chin, really?

While such activities can seem downright silly, sometimes silliness can be healing. Licensed Massage Therapist Michele Herling works to teach non-violence through touch in her non-profit organization, Compassionate Touch. Compassionate Touch has brought self-massage, chi gung, and even face dancing to the children of Bosnia.

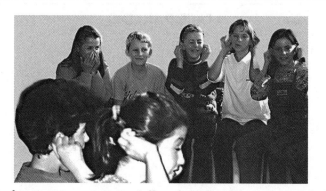

Kindergartners are especially adept face dancers, Michele
has discovered. (For more info, see RESOURCES)

MOVEMENT, THE NERVOUS SYSTEM, AND TRAUMA:

There is a strong relationship between the gunas, the currents, and the nervous system. Stone's Chart #17 in
Evolutionary Energy Charts is a vital resource here.

GUNA	Sattva	Rajas	Tamas
PRINCIPLE	Air	Fire	Water
NERVOUS SYSTEM	Parasympathetic nervous system	Sympathetic nervous system	Cerebral spinal fluid

(49)

There are techniques, knowingly or unknowingly, that
relate to the patterns of movement and healing found in the
currents. For example, EMDR, a popular method used mainly
by psychotherapists, initiates voluntary side-to-side movements in clients' eyes, or uses side-to-side touch on the
knees. Its aim is to access the nervous system to clear long-
held patterns of stress. This can be another way to work
with the transverse current.

Lee Cartwright of Santa Fe, New Mexico, has developed an intriguing system that expands EMDR practices into all three dimensions. He calls his work SCtD ⁽ᵀᴹ⁾ Meditations. It looks to be a promising way to both reframe and release trauma (see RESOURCES). Cartwright's hypothesis is that his system of movement, touch, and thought heal through their integration of the nervous system. My guess is that it also works with all three currents, part of its effectiveness. Its practices can be used with oneself or in a Polarity session.

In summary, these three currents are one potent gateway to life and healing, and may be a dynamic way to balance the doshas.

CHAPTER SYNOPSIS:

MOVEMENT:

Do you want to:

take a walk or run or stroll outside in the early morning?
or

play with Three Currents Chi Gung?
or

do some Polarity Yoga stretches?
or

do a SynergyDance with your currents?
or

smile: stretch those face muscles?

RESOURCES IN MOVEMENT:
BOOKS AND VIDEOS:

Alon, Ruthy, *Mindful Spontaneity: Lessons in the Feldenkrais Method*, specifically explores how this method can help a painful back. Wise woman.

Anderson, Bob, *Stretching*, very fine book, with warm-up routines for a wide range of activities.

Burger, Bruce, *Esoteric Anatomy*, has an excellent section on toe reading from a master of the art, p. 338-343.

Calais-Germain, Blandine, *Anatomy of Movement*, if you'd like to see what your bones and muscles are doing as you move, here's an accessible inside view. Fosters deeper understanding of physical structure, with many line drawing illustrations.

Cartwright, Lee, *SCtD (TM) Meditations: Transformational Tools for the Health Practitioner: An Introduction in Outline Form*, 1472 St. Francis Dr., Santa Fe, NM 87505, integrates movement, touch, and awareness in releasing trauma via all three dimensions.

Chakravarti, Sree, *A Healer's Journey*, a remarkable woman's journey in healing, see p. 197-202 for yoga for healing.

Chitty, Anna, *Energy Exercises* video, Polarity Press, 1721 Redwood Ave., Boulder, CO 80304, (303) 443-9847. Well-done Polarity Yoga video from an astute Polarity Therapy practitioner.

Chitty, John and Mary Louise Muller, *Energy Exercises: Easy Exercises for Health & Vitality* (book), 1990, Polarity Press, 1721 Redwood Ave., Boulder, CO 80304, (303) 443-9847. Includes appendices that key you into specific Polarity Yoga exercises for each element and guna. It also has a strong section on body reading of the face, torso and toes, and integrates the Educational Kinesiology wisdom of Paul and Gail Dennison in its approaches.

Dennison, Paul E. and Gail E., *Brain Gym: Simple Activities for Whole Brain Learning*, whimsical and effective methods for children and adults.

Desikachar, T.K.V., *The Heart of Yoga: Developing a Personal Practice*, an introduction to Viniyoga.

Francis, John, *Polarity Yoga: A Series of Self-Help Exercises*, the first published manual on this subject, is available through APTA.

Kraftsow, Gary, *Yoga for Wellness: Healing with the Timeless Teachings of Viniyoga*, includes many excellent programs of therapeutic yoga; sensible, clear.

Lee, Charmaine, Gong of Four (Charmaine Lee, Roger Piantadosi, et al), *SynergyDance* videotape, Grace Notes, 5207 Wisconsin Ave. NW, Washington DC, 20015, (800) 578-6678, this one hour videotape guides you in an easy to follow, dynamic dance through the elements.

Rawlinson, Ian, *Yoga for the West*, well-done manual of Viniyoga.

Sills, Franklyn, *The Polarity Process: Energy as a Healing Art*, includes much information about the currents, strong book for practitioners.

Stone, Randolph, all of his books, especially *Health Building: The Conscious Art of Living Well*, p. 130-187.

PROGRAMS:

Castellino Prenatal and Birth Trauma Therapy and Training, Raymond F. Castellino, DC, RPP, (805) 687-2897, 1105 N. Ontare Rd, Santa Barbara, CA, 93105-1937, SandraCAST@aol.com, does pioneering work integrating Polarity Therapy and early development; the program's primary focus is the training of professionals in the healing arts in their work with infants and young children.

Compassionate Touch, learning non-violence through touch, a project in the US and eastern Europe, c/o Michele Herling, LMT, 1967 Kiva St., Santa Fe, NM 87505-3314, (505) 982-0904.

ImpulseWork Process Seminars and Training Series, presents Dr. James Said, DC, ND, RPP and his unique understanding of energy medicine and the body, Energy Medicine Center of Petaluma, (707) 773-1133, or for registration, Sheila Donlan at (707) 775-3405.

Southwest Yoga Conference: there are many fine yoga conferences today, and this is one of the best, integrating Ayurveda and Yoga in its program offerings. It takes place annually in the Southwest, contact Julie Deife, P O Box 1932, Corrales, NM 87048, (505) 890-5133, email: info@southwestyoga.com, web page: www.southwestyoga.com.

SynergyDance and Healing Arts Center, 5207 Wisconsin Ave. NW, Washington DC, 20015, (800) 578-6678, web page: www.synergy-dance.com, Charmaine Lee, RPP offers programs in SynergyDance as well as SynergyDance Teacher Training.

III.

———•———

BREATH

The Experience of Prana, Tejas and Ojas.

"Prana is radiant energy."
STONE, *POLARITY THERAPY, VOL. I, BK. 1, P. 60*

Breath marks our entryway into this world; its departure signals our leaving. In the ancient traditions, breath is more than just air: it carries vital energy. This energy is called *prana* in Polarity Therapy and Ayurveda, and *chi* in Chinese medicine and acupuncture.

The skillful use of breath has been used for thousands of years in many traditions, to heal, to calm the mind, to come into union with the Source. As Stone pointed out, *"Prana is literally the 'Manna' from heaven. It cannot be stored, but must be gathered anew, every morning and every moment, with every breath. It is this radiant energy which keeps the body buoyant, vigorous and healthy."* (1)

Deep breathing delivered freely to every cell of our bodies is essential to health. If we are fortunate enough to breathe deeply automatically, this breath will carry prana where it is needed. If we are not so lucky, as evidenced by stiffness, stagnation, congestion, or depression, we need to make a conscious effort to breathe. And to open our respiratory channels.

Prana is carried on the three Polarity currents of the body, as well as through countless channels within the body, known as *srotas* or *nadis*. The yogis of India used breath in many ways. Generally taking a breath "in" is building, while breathing "out" is cleansing. One of the

simplest methods of *pranayama* is simply alternate breathing, or what could be called, "the cross-crawl of the brain".
It is a safe, effective way to calm the mind and increase the
absorption of prana to the brain, when done in moderation.
It is usually done immediately before meditation, to calm
the waters of the mind and to assist in going more deeply
into a still space.

PRANAYAMA

There are many ways to do pranayama. It is taught as a
healing science in and of itself. Breath can be used to calm
fire; warm air, earth, and water; or promote stronger
digestion; depending on the pattern you breath. The
alternate breathing I am most familiar with is a simple
one which calms the mind. Pranayama is done on an
empty stomach with a straight back and clear nostrils. If
you've got a cold, or you've just eaten, these are not times
to do pranayama.

You can begin with a gentle breath in and out of both
nostrils. Settle down and let yourself get comfortable
with a straight back. Take a breath into your chest
through both nostrils, block your right nostril with your
right thumb, and breath out, exhale, through the left nostril, pulling in your abdominal muscles from your pubic
bone as you do. This is the beginning of the cycle. Once
you've completely exhaled through that nostril, breath in
through the same nostril, the left one, letting your chest
expand. Now stop blocking the right nostril, block the left
one instead with your right forefinger, and breath out
through the right, letting your abdominal muscles gently
contract. Then breathe in through the right nostril into
your chest. This is one cycle of breath. You would go on
to exhale through your left, inhale through the left,
exhale through the right, inhale through the right.
Usually twelve cycles are done, just like the first one. To
begin, you might want to try it five or six times.

Pranayama

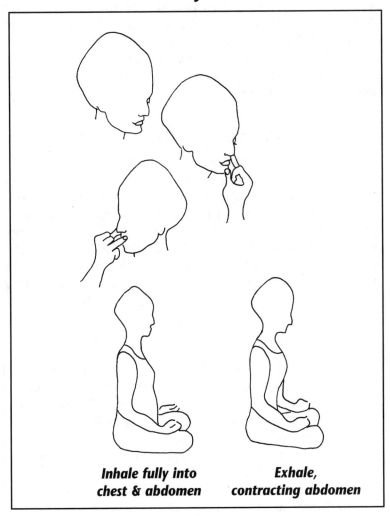

Inhale fully into chest & abdomen

Exhale, contracting abdomen

Science is beginning to substantiate the powerful effects of the breath. As Candace B. Pert, Ph.D., research professor in physiology and biophysics at Georgetown University Medical Center in Washington D.C., has observed: "There is a wealth of data showing that changes in the rate and depth of breathing produce changes in the quantity and kind of peptides that are released from the brain stem. And vice versa!

Virtually any peptide found anywhere else can be found in the respiratory center. This peptide substrate may provide the scientific rationale for the powerful healing effects of consciously controlled breath patterns." (2) These peptides influence immunity, mood, endurance, and other factors crucial to health, a potential biochemical link with the ancient concept of prana.

ABOUT PRANA AND BREATH:

Dr. Stone and many yogis have said plainly that breath, oxygen, and prana are not synonymous. Breath is a carrier for oxygen, and oxygen is a carrier for prana. Without breath or oxygen, prana cannot be absorbed into our respiratory systems. Prana is an alive and easily dispersed energy that can be found in fresh air, running water, and fresh food. It is not found in bottled water or oxygen delivered in tanks. We must get it through our own effort of breathing and eating: this is how this energy feeds us. (3)

PLAYING WITH BREATH AND PRANA

We are all at different points in our journey with breath and prana. Some of us benefit greatly from the conscious breathing used in pranayama, some meditation processes, or yoga practice. Conscious inhalation and exhalation are specifically used to clear prana in ida, pingala, and sushumna as a preliminary to some meditation techniques. For others of us, conscious breathing practices can become habitual and routine, trapping us in particular ways of thinking and perceiving the world. If this could be you, take a moment and let go: invite the breath of this next moment to breathe you, and feel what happens.

In SynergyDance, it is suggested that you let yourself breathe naturally as you move, with the idea that you are taking in and distributing prana with each breath and movement. As a way to directly experience this, imagine

---

breathing through your feet, inviting the energy of the earth into your toes and soles. How does this feel? When you think about it, you are really taking in prana, energy, rather than literal oxygen as you do this. (4)

You can trust that you will find appropriate ways to play with breath and prana suited to you.

GETTING SERIOUS ABOUT BREATH AND DIGESTION

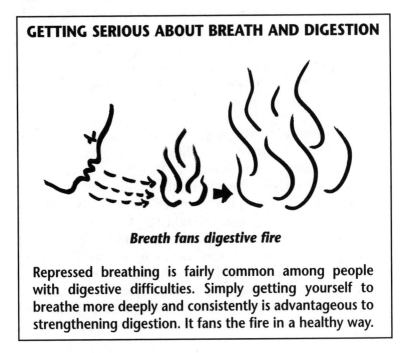

Breath fans digestive fire

Repressed breathing is fairly common among people with digestive difficulties. Simply getting yourself to breathe more deeply and consistently is advantageous to strengthening digestion. It fans the fire in a healthy way.

Usually breath is the focus, because that is our main way to gather prana. And yet there is another way to accumulate prana, and that is through well-absorbed fresh food. The nose and the colon are our gateways for prana! In other words, prana must come in to our bodies through very earthy entryways. If the sinuses or gut are congested, we will pick up less prana. If our air or our food is of poor quality, there will be less prana available in it to be absorbed.

Once we take in this vital energy, it must be circulated. Here, the strength of the heart and blood is crucial. If we are anemic or have an over-worked heart, we will be delivering less prana to every cell. Exercise, building the blood, strengthening the heart are all keys in these situations to enhancing overall vitality.

Stone summarized the dance between breath and body in the following way: *"When the body is in good health there is a natural balance and relationship between the breath of life and its conveyor, the blood stream as a fluid, and its rhythmic beat through the central pump called the heart." "When there is insufficient life breath in the body the result is unresolved residues called blood sludge, which are deposited in the body tissues."* (5)

Many disorders, including the fungus *Candida* and the disease of cancer, thrive in conditions of lowered oxygen in the tissues and prana in the cells. Once prana is circulated, it affects every tissue, increasing its vitality and efficiency. To give one example: on the esoteric level, it is said that when prana is abundant, calcium stays in solution more easily, creating strong flexible bones and joints. When prana becomes low, calcium moves into a solid and less available form, contributing to arthritis and bone pain. (6) While this might sound wild initially, you can experiment with it yourself. Begin to notice whether breath and freedom of movement have any connections for you.

WHAT WE MIGHT BE:

A few years ago, I was attending a powwow and parade with a friend up in Jicarilla Apache country. I noticed a beautiful old woman hurrying across the blacktop main street just before the parade began, dodging the excited kids, dogs, soft drink and hat vendors with adept skill. What struck me was how incredibly fluid her movements were, for someone who looked fairly old. I asked my friend, who was in her early sixties, about her. "Oh, yes, that's

Maggie. My mother took photographs of her and her three children when I was young," she replied in a matter of fact way. This woman, so easy in her body, was a contemporary of my friend's mother, long since dead! She had to be in her eighties or nineties, yet she moved like someone in her twenties. Whatever she was doing, she knew how to accumulate prana easily and well.

THE BALANCE OF PRANA, TEJAS AND OJAS:

We can support our supply of vital energy in mundane simple ways, like breathing more deeply, maintaining clear lungs and digestive tract, eating fresh food. Or building up our heart and blood through exercise and kindness. Why is prana important? Besides keeping us supple, healthy and contented, it is THE energy so frequently discussed in Polarity Therapy. In other words, the more prana available to you, the faster and easier all of this Polarity work proceeds.

And yet you can have too much of a good thing. In Ayurveda and Yoga, the subtle energies of prana are usually considered in conjunction with two other subtle energies, *tejas,* and *ojas.* Polarity Therapy is definitely an activity in which one can apply an understanding of all three of these essences. While prana is our subtle breath, our life force, our chi, tejas is our creative fire. And ojas is our vital moist energy cushion, roughly equivalent to a healthy aura or strong, intact energy field within and around the physical body.

Dr. Stone's published writings describe prana and yet do not go into ojas or tejas by name, although he seemed aware of them energetically. For example, the following passage from *Health Building* (7) describes one way to rebuild what in Ayurveda would be called ojas: *"The electromagnetic fields will balance themselves as a rule, if given a chance Nature's way. Quieting the emotions by faith, hope, and love is most helpful. Water cleanses and rest restores weak-*

*ened magnetic fields, and makes us think; which alone can
remove many a kink."*

The practice of Polarity Therapy stimulates the flow of
prana. As prana moves, we can feel exhilarated, joyous,
light, clear. Ojas acts as a container and nourishment for
both prana and tejas. If ojas is strong, as the container for
prana, this joy can be integrated into our bodies and lives,
creating greater health and a sense of well being. Ojas also
stimulates immunity, strengthening our defenses and our
ability to respond effectively to changes in our environments and lives.

However, if ojas is weak, it is a bit like having thin top-
soil or a container that is too small, or leaks. You're trying
to grow these beautiful healthy plants, prana and tejas, and
yet they get to this certain point, the limits of their container, and they begin to struggle, like plants in poor soil. In
this case, if prana is increased through Polarity Therapy
work, the exhilarating experience is likely to be fleeting. In
the worst of extremes, such a situation might set off tempo-
rary nervous discharges or a kundalini crisis. These are not
conditions I want to help create, so we can explore here
how to prevent such difficulties. Understanding more about
these three vital energies can help enormously.

As prana flows through our subtle bodies, as well as our
more obvious physical cells, it flows through the chakras
and can activate *kundalini.* Kundalini literally means
"obstruction" in Sanskrit. (8) As obstructions are cleared in
our chakras' flows, energy can go rise up the body. This can
feel wonderful or uncomfortable, depending on our experience and perceptions.

It seems important for those of us working with Polarity
as well as spiritual practice to have some understanding of
this. Before we begin to build prana substantially, whether
through Polarity Therapy or pranayama, we need to build
ojas, because ojas acts as a safe and steady container for the
increasing prana. Healthy ojas helps keep prana grounded

and moving effectively, without dissipation. It also nurtures tejas, our creative imagination and energy.

How does one build ojas? Adequate rest, good night sleep, gentle devotional practices, pure nourishing food, and enough fluids are essential. Rest by water, especially flowing water, particularly waterfalls, is a time-honored way. These are valuable for anyone, especially those with a compromised immune system, which indicates reduced ojas. I'm not sure I can emphasize enough how helpful rest in conjunction with appropriate meditation can be. In *Charaka Samhita*, an ancient Ayurvedic text, a good night's sleep is called *bhutadhatri*: "that (which) nurses all beings, sleep caused by the nature of the night". (9)

How to reduce ojas? Overwork, worry, excess stimulation (such as cities, TV, loud noises, and excessive demands), excessive travel, excessive physical or mental or emotional output, not enough nourishing foods and fluids, not enough time for rest and nurturing spiritual practice. What feels like excessive stimulation to an introverted person may simply feel like normal, comfortable stimulation for another more extroverted individual, so it is important to recognize our own limits and needs. When we're fried, we're fried, whether it looks like we "ought" to be or not!

The doshas we explored earlier in chapter 1, Vata, Pitta, and Kapha, interact with prana, tejas, and ojas. In fact, some Ayurvedic practitioners consider the latter energies subtler expressions of the doshas, that is, prana relates in some ways to Vata, tejas to Pitta, and ojas to Kapha. Yet there is a crucial difference between the doshas and these subtler energies. When the doshas get out of balance, either too much or too little of any dosha, the body struggles. And yet, with the subtler energies, we can't have too much ojas, to my way of understanding. The more ojas around us, the more health, calm, and peace of mind we experience. And tejas and prana can increase then, too, which is considered favorable, balanced with generous ojas.

The doshas interact with these subtler energies in specific ways. Vata (our airy dosha) can accumulate in excess under the same kinds of stressful conditions, which deplete ojas. Excess Vata can literally begin to dry up our moist cushion of ojas, on an energetic level, when we overwork or eat improperly. Then if prana gets high during Polarity Therapy or with too much pranayama or lots of chanting or breath work, we can have nervous discharges.

How can we prevent this? Acknowledge we need rest, space, fluids, food, love. This includes receiving these before, during, and after workshops and intense work times. Gardening and other unstructured times in nature can be good ways to build ojas. (10) For many of us, it is simply maintaining a sane balance between input and output.

There are also spiritual practices which simultaneously build up all three energies, which is a favorable state in which to be. (11)

As prana begins to flow, we have a chance to see our chakras in a new light.

UNDERSTANDING PRANA, TEJAS, AND OJAS

When present:	You will see quality of:
Prana (life-force)	mental interest and aliveness
Tejas (inner radiance)	creative enthusiasm and heightened perception, brilliance in the energy field
Ojas (primal vigor)	being at peace with oneself, patience, contentment, satisfaction, endurance

In terms of the esoteric anatomy of Yoga and Ayurveda, all three of these subtle energies are supported by reproductive fluid, which generates ojas. There is more specific information about this and how to build your own physical reproductive fluids in chapter 7. Taoist practices, as well as

Ayurvedic and Chinese medicine, have historically had deep appreciation for the value of regenerative and rejuvenative practices. While cleansing is important, building is, too. If we are run-down, our ability to help ourselves or others, or to explore spiritually, suffers. If we are to work with energy healing on any kind of regular basis, the generation and conservation of vital energy is essential to understand.

Ojas is the fuel for tejas and the grounding for prana. If ojas increases, so can prana and tejas. If ojas is depleted, prana and tejas suffer.

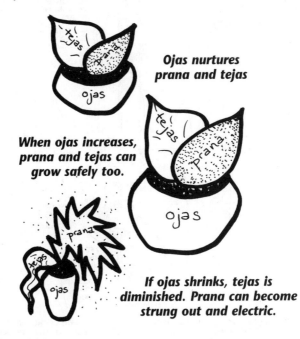

Ojas nurtures prana and tejas

When ojas increases, prana and tejas can grow safely too.

If ojas shrinks, tejas is diminished. Prana can become strung out and electric.

THE FIVE PRANAS

Vata dosha is sub-divided into five categories of vata, called prana, udana, samana, vyana, and apana. Dr. Stone in some of his writings referred to these as the five pranas. In one chart included in *Polarity Therapy*, Stone correlates the long lines running along the soles of the feet with the five pranas. Physically working along these long lines on the bottoms of the feet is another way to help balance Vata and stimulate a freer flow of prana to the body. (12)

CHART NO. **2**   CHART OF THE SUBTLE PRANA CURRENTS IN THE
HUMAN BODY AND THEIR CHAKRAS AS WHIRLING
PRIMARY <u>FUNCTIONAL</u> CENTERS OF ENERGY.

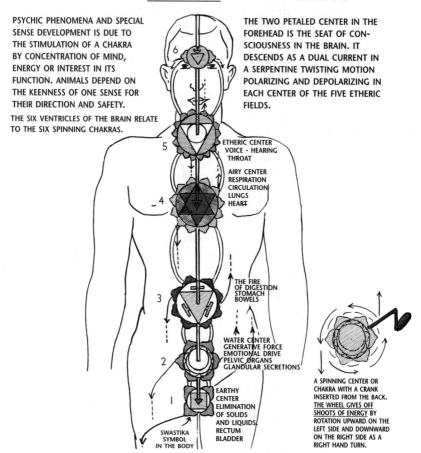

PSYCHIC PHENOMENA AND SPECIAL SENSE DEVELOPMENT IS DUE TO THE STIMULATION OF A CHAKRA BY CONCENTRATION OF MIND, ENERGY OR INTEREST IN ITS FUNCTION. ANIMALS DEPEND ON THE KEENNESS OF ONE SENSE FOR THEIR DIRECTION AND SAFETY.

THE SIX VENTRICLES OF THE BRAIN RELATE TO THE SIX SPINNING CHAKRAS.

THE TWO PETALED CENTER IN THE FOREHEAD IS THE SEAT OF CONSCIOUSNESS IN THE BRAIN. IT DESCENDS AS A DUAL CURRENT IN A SERPENTINE TWISTING MOTION POLARIZING AND DEPOLARIZING IN EACH CENTER OF THE FIVE ETHERIC FIELDS.

ETHERIC CENTER
VOICE - HEARING
THROAT

AIRY CENTER
RESPIRATION
CIRCULATION
LUNGS
HEART

THE FIRE
OF DIGESTION
STOMACH
BOWELS

WATER CENTER
GENERATIVE FORCE
EMOTIONAL DRIVE
PELVIC ORGANS
GLANDULAR SECRETIONS

EARTHY
CENTER
ELIMINATION
OF SOLIDS
AND LIQUIDS.
RECTUM
BLADDER

SWASTIKA
SYMBOL
IN THE BODY

A SPINNING CENTER OR CHAKRA WITH A CRANK INSERTED FROM THE BACK. <u>THE WHEEL GIVES OFF SHOOTS OF ENERGY</u> BY ROTATION UPWARD ON THE LEFT SIDE AND DOWNWARD ON THE RIGHT SIDE AS A RIGHT HAND TURN.

THE CENTER LINE THROUGH THE BODY IS THE LOCATION OF THE PATH OF THE ULTRA-SONIC ENERGY SUBSTANCE AS THE PRIMARY LIFE CURRENT AND THE CORE OF BEING. IT FLOWS THROUGH THE SIXTH VENTRICLE OF THE BRAIN AND THE SPINAL CORD. IT HAS FIVE STEPDOWN CENTERS BELOW THE BRAIN FOR THE SPECIALIZATION OF FUNCTIONS WHICH WE CALL THE LAWS OF NATURE FOR MOTION, LIFE AND THE PRESERVATION OF THE SPECIES. THESE CENTERS IN THE FIVE OVAL ETHERIC FIELDS ARE THE CORE OF THE WIRELESS ANATOMY OF THE FINEST PARTICLES OF MATTER KNOWN AS CHAKRAS OR LOTUSES. AS THEY WHIRL IN A RIGHT HAND DIRECTION FROM THE BACK, EACH OF THE FIVE CENTERS GIVES OFF ONE WAVE OF ITS SPECIAL QUALITY OF VIBRATORY ENERGY FLOWING AS AN ELECTRO-MAGNETIC CIRCUIT TO EACH FINGER AND TOE. IN THIS MANNER THE SENSORY AND THE FIVE MOTOR SENSES ARE CREATED AND FUNCTION IN THE BODY.

The Subtle Prana Currents (chakras). Reprinted from Dr. Randolph Stone, *Polarity Therapy*, vol. I, bk. 2, p. 9, with gracious permission by CRCS Publications.

CHART OF THE SUBTLE PRANA CURRENTS IN THE HUMAN BODY AND THEIR CHAKRAS AS WHIRLING PRIMARY <u>FUNCTIONAL</u> CENTERS OF ENERGY.

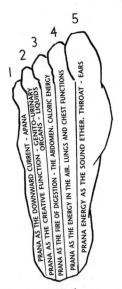

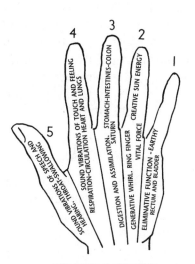

MIND AND PRANA (LIFE BREATH) FUNCTION THRU THE FIELDS OF MATTER AND ITS CENTERS

THESE ENERGY LINES ARE PURELY FUNCTIONAL AND PSYCHOLOGICAL AS LONGITUDINAL INFLUENCE ARISING FROM THE CHAKRAS AND FORMING THE FIVE SENSORY AND THE FIVE MOTOR CURRENTS FLOWING THROUGH THE BODY TO EACH DIGIT OF THE HANDS AND FEET. IN THE TREATMENT OF FUNCTIONAL BLOCKS OR DISTURBANCE OF THE FIVE SENSES THESE AREAS ARE USEFUL WHEN THE PHYSIOLOGY IS MOSTLY INVOLVED.

THE HAND IS THE SAME FUNCTIONAL NEUTER POLE AS THE FOOT IS THE NEGATIVE POLE. CHART NO. 4 GIVES DEFINITE REGIONAL ANATOMI-CAL LOCATIONS FOR AFFECTING STRUCTURAL CHANGES BY MANIPULATION OR PRESSURE ON DEFINITE REFLEX AREAS.

The Subtle Prana Currents (hands & feet). Reprinted from Dr. Randolph Stone, *Polarity Therapy*, vol. I, bk. 2, p. 9, with gracious permission by CRCS Publications.

MAKING PRANA OR CHI TANGIBLE:

For some of us, tangible physical proofs are needed to persuade us that these subtle energies are real. We are living in times when exactly this is becoming possible. In one fascinating series of experiments, Western-trained physicist Zang-Hee Cho has used MRI, magnetic resonance imaging, "to provide scientific proof of how acupuncture works in the brain." With shifting patterns of response in the brain to point stimulation in other parts of the body, Dr. Cho believes his experiments may also be providing demonstrations of chi (prana), yin (centripetal energy), and yang (centrifugal energy). (13)

PLANETARY OJAS:

The planet also has an energy field, and a store of ojas. The last fifty to one hundred years of intensive industrialization and chemical discharge into the environment has put major strains on the energy cushion of the earth.

For the longevity and health of all creatures on the planet, human habits need to shift radically. If we continue to drive automobiles, fly, and dump chemicals in the current ways and rates, the immunity of all those who follow us is inevitably compromised. (14)

HEART IS THE SEAT OF OJAS:

In Ayurveda, the heart is the seat of ojas in the human body. The heart is also where subtle prana makes its home. Keeping a clear heart nurtures both ojas and prana within. (15)

Heart, the Seat of Ojas

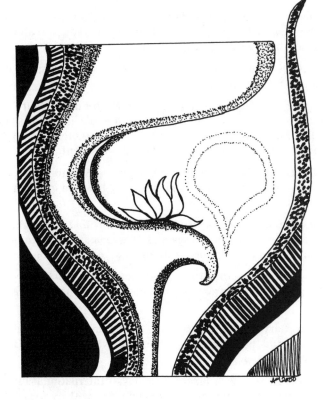

CHAPTER SYNOPSIS:

BREATH:

Do you want to:

breathe?

breathe deeply?

work with pranayama?

nurture your vital reserves through rest and meditation?

absorb prana or chi through fresh vital food?

support your capacity to absorb prana with exercise and
kindness?

RESOURCES IN BREATH:

Buhrman, Sarasvati, "Ayurveda and the Breath" in *Yoga International*, May 1997, as well as subsequent articles in later issues, is an excellent discussion from a skilled practitioner.

Chakravarti, Sree, *A Healer's Journey*, includes a fine section on "The Prana and Self-Healing", p. 191-196.

Farhi, Donna, *The Breathing Book: Good Health and Vitality Through Essential Breath Work*: this yogini is interested in the free flow of breath throughout the body. She skillfully explores how to do this physically with conscious awareness and movement.

Frawley, David, "Balancing Subtle Energy: The Spiritual Dimension of Ayurveda", in *Yoga International*, Jan./Feb. 1996, an excellent discussion of prana, tejas, and ojas.

Frawley, David, *Yoga & Ayurveda: Self-Healing and Self-Realization*, a stimulating exploration of yoga and Ayurveda and their connections, with discussion about prana, tejas and ojas on p. 87-103.

Johari, Harish, *Breath, Mind, and Consciousness*, Destiny Books, Rochester, VT, 1989, provides an in-depth yogic perspective on this topic.

Kraftsow, Gary, *Yoga for Wellness*, p. 7–12, includes a great discussion of breath and pranayama, clear and practical, from a fine yoga teacher.

Swami Rama, *Science of Breath*, Himalayan International Institute of Yoga Science and Philosophy, Honesdale, PA, 1981, is a small gem of a book from a master of the subject.

See also Notes to Practitioners, in Appendix, about prana and ojas.

IV.

STILLNESS

Sattva. Dr. Stone on Listening Meditation and
the Experience of the Step-down of Energy.

"The finer possibilities awaken when the individual is ready!"
STONE, HEALTH BUILDING, P. 106.

SATTVA: clear, centered.

Dr. Stone was profoundly interested in the spiritual life,
and strongly believed that "tuning in with God" was the
highest priority in health and healing. He explored the mys-
tic traditions of Sufism, the Rosicrucian path, the Kabbalah,
Christianity, and Hinduism in depth, ultimately settling
into the practice of Sant Mat with his teacher Charan Singh
in India. Given the fruits of Stone's wide ranging spiritual
explorations, it appears to me that any spiritual practice
which can be used to move into stillness and a deeper alignment with spirit is compatible and supportive of the
practice of energy healing.

Much of the information Dr. Stone shared was gathered
while, as he put it, he was "burning the midnight oil". It is
possible to confirm for yourself, inside yourself, many of his
discoveries in meditation, with patient application. As he
put it, *"Tuning in with the Infinite is a practical idea, if
applied and understood."* (1)

He described a particular practice which can be taken literally with powerful results. *"The secret to learn here is for
man's (sic) consciousness to remain still in the CENTER OF
BEING, in its eternal essence. Then things will right themselves. The Holy Bible states this in simple terms: 'Be still,
and know that I am God.' (PSALM 46:10)* (2) He maintained

that this practice of stillness freed up the Central Energy, the core, *sushumna*, and was potently restorative to health.

Consequently, the intention of this chapter is to support you in your own spiritual practice, whatever it might be. We will be exploring here Stone's perspectives on the experience of stillness to strengthen your meditations. There are many other valuable practices; in my experience, the following process seems to be helpful both as a preliminary practice and for meditators with more experience.

A PRACTICE OF COMING INTO STILLNESS

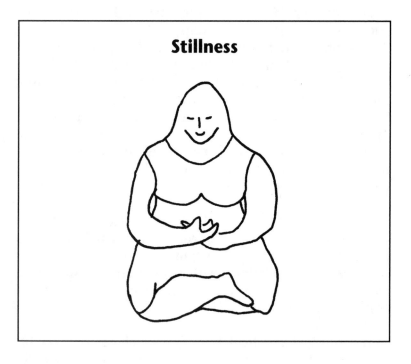

Stillness

You may already have a practice with which you work, or no. If you are interested in exploring a method directly related to Dr. Stone's Polarity practice, here is one possibility.

Sit quietly and comfortably, with a relaxed, straight back. You can ask for the highest good, offering yourself as a vehicle for this work. Begin to quiet your mind. A series of simple alternate breathing can be very useful for this, see Pranayama, p. 112. As you quiet your mind, begin to listen your way into your core, the central channel. Simply listen, ignoring your own mental comments, just as you would if you were listening intently to another person in a conversation. Here you are listening your way into the silence. This may take many times, or it may come quickly, we are each different. It is possible to listen your way into an experience of deep silence that is palpable. For me it sometimes feels like entering a great wood of ancient trees, that kind of presence; you may associate the silence with something else entirely, or better yet, nothing at all. There is nothing to imagine or visualize or chant or do, simply listen. Your intention is to listen. Just keep listening. Allow the silence to nourish you, deep within.

For people familiar with craniosacral work, the experience is quite similar to that moment when you move into still point and stay there. When your mind starts to get restless and wander, stop there in that moment. If you want, you can offer up the fruits of your focus for the benefit of all beings. Stop there until the next time you want to do this.

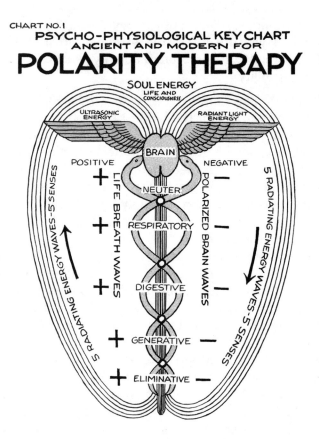

Chart #1: Polarity Therapy. Reprinted from Dr. Randolph Stone, *Polarity Therapy*, vol. I, bk. 3, p. 26, with gracious permission by CRCS Publications.

OPENING TO THE STEP-DOWN OF ENERGY

After you have done the practice of stillness for awhile, as you open to the silence, the divine within, you may notice sensations of opening or focus. These may occur somewhere in your head, throat or neck. Simply allow that to happen. It may continue downward around and in you. If this feels comfortable to you, you can invite the energy in, make it welcome. It may proceed downward through the center of your chest, to your solar plexus, the lower abdomen, the perineal floor. This is one direct experience of what Dr. Stone

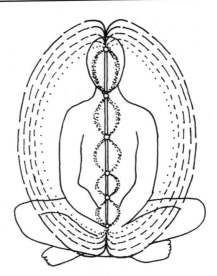

called "the step-down of energy" from spirit inside to our physical form. Opening to this experience can be a practice of communion, spiritual nourishment, and rejuvenation.

Stone once observed, "Truly, bliss resides at the very core of perfect equilibrium, out of which the creation was manifested. It is also present at the very core of man's being, like the stillness in the depths of the oceans." (3) Dr. Stone was a remarkably subtle being, his preacher-style notwithstanding. You can take this statement, as well as many others he made, literally. Let yourself discover what he was talking about here. (4) Most of his suggestions are simple practices; it just takes commitment, intention and focus to discover their dynamics for yourself.

Note: this is one example of a receptive, centripetal process.

CHAPTER SYNOPSIS:

STILLNESS:

Do you want to:

focus into stillness?

RESOURCES IN STILLNESS:

Especially valuable here are the two volumes of Stone's *Polarity Therapy*, particularly Stone, *Polarity Therapy*, vol. I, bk. 1, p. 47, and vol. I, bk. 3, p. 5, as well as Stone, *Health Building*, p. 26.

Tarchin, *Meditative First Aid: A Doorway to Health*, Wangapeka Books, P.O. Box 80-141, Green Bay, Auckland, New Zealand, a small manual of fresh starts.

V.

NOURISHMENT: HEALING WITH FOOD

Exploring how the Gunas Relate to
Food and its Preparation.

*"The selection of food is according to each one's tempera-
ment. The __mind__ must be satisfied with the food and drink."*
STONE, *POLARITY THERAPY*, VOL. *I, BK. 3, P. 111*

*"Every blade of grass has the power to attract what it
needs from the earth, the water, the air and the warm
sun rays, to make its own vibratory pattern in life. All
life—vegetable, animal and human—shares alike in this
provision of these four polarized energies in their flow."*
STONE, *POLARITY THERAPY*, VOL. *I, BK. 1, P. 15*

In our day here together, we've gotten up and done some
early morning routines, moved, breathed, and meditated. It's
time for nourishment.

ABOUT NOURISHMENT:

Life is precious. We live on a planet whose key resources
are being rapidly diminished. Many of us on this planet
don't get enough to eat to survive, while others of us struggle with not being able to say "no" to too much. There is a
flood of energy around food, what to eat, what is enough,
what is OK. My primary intention in this chapter is to invite
each of us to move toward inner healing around food, in
whatever way has meaning for us. We are each of us so different; I cannot realistically suggest one diet for everyone,
or even three or four basic types, although I do offer some
rough guidelines like this later in this chapter.

I have been a therapeutic nutritionist for twenty-five years now. In that time, I have seen many kinds of food therapies help individuals, and some harm them. My focus is to create as much healing and as little damage as possible. Initially I became interested in Ayurveda as a Western nutritionist working with people dealing with cancer. At that time, I was searching for answers as to why fresh vegetable juice fasts really helped some people heal, and yet only seemed to weaken others. Ayurveda offered helpful perspectives on individualized healing.

Ethically, I've been attracted to vegetarian diets, and I've written several Ayurvedic cookbooks with a vegetarian focus. Both Ayurveda and Polarity Therapy can be easily practiced from a vegetarian perspective, and there is a lot of support for this from practitioners in both fields. And yet, having worked with many people over these two to three decades, now I am more interested in creating nourishment plans that suit individual needs, than to promote any particular ideology around food. I want to explore further why sometimes one food approach is useful, and in other circumstances, it is not.

With this in mind, these are the questions I've found useful in helping people arrive at nourishment plans that work.

ASSESSING YOUR OWN NOURISHMENT

Is what I eat easily digestible for me?

Does it support my health and well being?

Does it help create a calm, grounded center inside me?

Is it ethical, from my perspective?

If I were to change anything in the way I eat or drink
now to meet my needs more effectively,
what would it be?

These are the basic opening questions. For many of us this is enough, and there is no need to go further. For others of us, nourishment is a complex and bedeviling topic that touches us not only physically, but also emotionally, mentally, and spiritually. I would invite you to move into as deep a harmony with the world around you as you are willing to hold, as you answer the following questions:

A DEEPER ASSESSMENT OF NOURISHMENT

What feeds me now?   What smells?
                       What tastes?
                       What sights?
                       What touch?
                       What sounds?

Do I need more or less of any of these?

Do I yearn for more subtle or blatant nourishment?

Am I willing to let myself have this?

Do I want to share the nourishment I receive with others?
  With my family and friends?
  With my community?
  With the larger community of people on this earth?
  With the larger community of animals, plants,
  beings on this earth?

How could I do this, manageably and practically?

Am I willing to do this?

When I went to India in the early 1980's, I had a strong and unsettling experience. I realized that I had been starving all my life without knowing it, and that something in India fed me deeply. Clearly, not everyone feels this way. And yet for the first time in my life, I felt fed. It was a myriad of sounds and smells and people. It was the blatant unashamed devotion that people had at temple, the permission to dive into spirit and be fed. It was harder for me to come back from India than to go: I had to face the sterility of experiences like American malls, or what sounded like empty agendas on the popular media. Many travelers have had similar experiences, returning from a place they love, or a region that has seized their hearts, not always easily. Each of us needs something, inside and outside, to thrive. For many of us it won't be a trip to a foreign country, but something else: something as simple as a waterfall, a loved one, work that matters, a particular spiritual practice. I want to encourage you in finding what truly nourishes you.

These are the questions and issues that mean the most to me. The rest of what follows here is information that can be used to support your nourishment, if you desire more details about food and healing as they relate to Ayurveda and Polarity Therapy.

HABIT AND FOOD:

In Ayurveda there is the concept of *okasatmya*. Essentially okasatmya suggest that if our bodies are accustomed to a particular dietary regime, they will tolerate it surprisingly well, more than might be predicted by any nutritionist or healer. In the West we have a similar concept, embodied in the expression, "If it isn't broken, don't fix it."

Often the ways our families and communities have eaten are imprinted into our individual nourishment patterns far more deeply than we appreciate. This can be a positive source of strength and grounding on a day-to-day basis.

When our customary or habitual ways of eating no longer work for us, then is the time to look at the Ayurvedic idea of *satmya*. Satmya is becoming accustomed to that which is healing for us. When those three eggs every day for two decades cause our cholesterol to climb dangerously, satmya is beginning to cut back on the number of eggs we eat each week. When the usual skipping of meals results in shakiness, headaches, and low blood sugar rather than our usual blithe good health, satmya is learning how to remember to eat regular meals rich in protein and whole grain, when we first become hungry.

A good deal of information about food is presented in these three chapters, sometimes with widely varying perspectives or agendas. You can use what you like of these, always feeling free to return to okasatmya, that to which you are accustomed. And when illness or unpleasant consequences approach, you can also learn satmya, the way that is healing for you.

POLARITY FOOD PROCESSES:

In Polarity Therapy, Dr. Stone recommended three dietary processes, the Purifying diet, the Health Building diet and the Gourmet Vegetarian diet. Each was used for different purposes; all were vegetarian.

PURIFYING: The purifying diet is a strongly alkalizing diet, designed to clear out waste. It is not intended as a maintenance diet to be used for months on end, for most people. It is excellent for cleansing. It includes: fresh fruit and vegetables, both raw and cooked; sprouts: of seeds, grains, and legumes; soaked almonds in moderation; avocado in moderation, raw honey, herbs and spices; cold-pressed oils, except corn oil (it can inhibit the thyroid). Polarity tea is used often and Vitality liver flushes are usually done first thing every morning.

No salt is used with the food, to maximize the cleansing effects of the purifying process. Taken internally, salt is a builder, and has the effect of holding water as well as toxins in the system. Whereas salt used externally in salt rubs or baths is cleansing. It will attract the water and toxins out of the body. So you can use as much salt as you like, outside of your body, just don't put it in your mouth in this process.

HEALTH BUILDING: The health building diet was created as a maintenance kind of program which is especially easy on the liver, good clean "fuel". It can be used before or after a purifying regime, to ease your way into and out of cleansing, or as a maintenance program if your health has been compromised. It can be excellent in working with acute or chronic hepatitis, sluggish liver, impaired digestion, heart disease, or cancer.

The health building diet can also be used as a gentle cleansing program if you've been living the high life. Or it can serve as a moderate relatively low-calorie building program, which is likely to promote weight loss, if that's what you are after. It includes: every food in the purifying process, plus unheated milk products, potatoes, legumes and whole grains, raw nuts and seeds, mushrooms, salt, nutritional yeast, miso, umeboshi plum paste, and tamari. Strong focus is placed on appropriate food combinations to maximize ease of digestion. Heated oils and fats are avoided on the health building diet to spare the liver. Optimally, your biggest meal is eaten at noon, with a lighter meal at suppertime to make best use of your digestive fire.

VEGETARIAN GOURMET: Dr. Stone understood that not everyone wanted to wear a halo at all times. The gourmet vegetarian diet was created for those times when you've had it with building your health and sanity, and want to play a bit. It is a lacto-vegetarian plan that encompasses all of the foods in the purifying and health building processes, plus cooked dairy, heated oils, ghee, and sautéed foods. It omits eggs, to enhance the sattvic qualities of the process. (1) The easiest pitfall in the gourmet veggie plan is to get into sweets more than you might need; it's wise to go easy on concentrated sweets here. If you find yourself craving sweets, check to be sure you're getting enough protein and whole grains.

It is important to note here that Randolph Stone had a pioneering sense about natural foods, as unique as his approach to bodywork. Decades before it became popular to do, he urged the use of organic produce, and the avoidance of aluminum in cookware. (2)

POLARITY FOOD PROCESSES

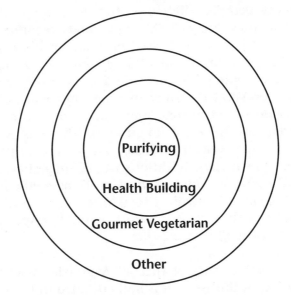

Purifying

Health Building

Gourmet Vegetarian

Other

PURIFYING includes: fresh fruit and vegetables, both raw and cooked, sprouted seeds, sprouted grains, and sprouted legumes, sweet potatoes, soaked almonds (in moderation), avocado (in moderation), raw honey, herbs and spices, cold-pressed oils (except corn), Polarity tea, and Vitality liver flush. No salt is used, to maximize cleansing.

HEALTH BUILDING includes everything in the Purifying process, plus: unheated milk products, potatoes, legumes and whole grains, raw nuts and seeds, mushrooms, salt, nutritional yeast. Miso, umeboshi plum paste, and tamari are part of a Health-building diet. Appropriate food combinations are emphasized, to maximize ease of digestion. Heated oils and fats are avoided on the Health-building diet, to spare the liver. If you can, having your biggest meal at noon and a lighter meal at suppertime makes the best use of your digestive fire.

VEGETARIAN GOURMET includes everything above, plus "all lacto-vegetarian foods", prepared with love and care (sattva). This includes cooked dairy, heated oils, ghee, sauteed foods, and many foods in an Ayurvedic food plan. No eggs are used, to enhance the sattvic qualities of the process. It's wise to go easy on concentrated sweets here. (1)

OTHER includes all other foods imaginable, including eggs, fish, poultry, red meat. "Other" foods are not used when doing Polarity Food Processes.

AYURVEDA AND FOOD:

While vegetarian diets are often used for healing in Ayurveda, they are not the only foods recommended. Vegetarian food is considered optimal for cleansing, as well as a good builder of ojas, our energy cushion. Yet there are exceptions to this rule. For example, if the air element (or Vata) is strong in a person's make-up, and that person has struggled long and hard on a balanced vegetarian diet with no tangible health benefits, or, in fact, is getting weaker or sicker, an Ayurvedic program based on the ancient traditions would suggest adding in foods like chicken soup or meat broth as medicine. The ancient Ayurvedic medical texts often used meat therapeutically, with a clear sense of personal responsibility for this choice. (3)

This is not to suggest that all Ayurvedic practitioners think alike on this issue; it is hotly debated in these times. Ayurvedic practitioners with a strong Hindu or Jain background wish to honor their traditions and beliefs, and use exclusively vegetarian diets, as Randolph Stone did in the development of Polarity Energetic Nutrition. Other Ayurvedic practitioners, regardless of religious tradition, see vegetarian diet as a way to honor life and support the planet, besides being a practical, personally healthy choice. Still other Ayurvedic practitioners see the need to return to the ancient recommendations, which included meat as medicine, when a person's health suffers with a vegetarian program. In my experience as a Western and Ayurvedic nutritionist over the last twenty-five years, I have come to appreciate that each of us has different needs, and I see all these views as valid. I sometimes recommend fish, poultry, or organic red meat therapeutically, honoring the being from which that medicine comes.

So what works for you? Hopefully this chapter, plus the two which follow about cleansing and building, will give you enough orientation that you can begin to decide for yourself. Western nutrition is notorious in our times for its changeable recommendations. While it is based on the latest scientific findings, scrapped together into the best patchwork quilt we nutritionists can weave, the beauty of both Ayurvedic and Polarity nutrition is that they are founded on more timeless principles. Whether they are effective for you remains to be seen. This information is no substitute for your own common sense and practical experience.

AYURVEDA: THE GUNAS IN FOOD:

To begin, it is important to consider that working with the gunas in food is particularly potent. Just as sattva, rajas and tamas play a role in mind and action, they also are active principles in food. This is described fairly clearly in Ayurvedic nutrition. Sattvic foods promote a clear, neutral, sattvic state of mind. Pure, fresh vegetarian foods, cooked or raw, make up the bulk of this category. How food is prepared is also important, as the energy we hold when we cook is conveyed to each person who eats it. That is why it is said that it is important to cook with love if you want to eat sattvic food. A fresh tempeh burger grilled with fury (rajas) is rajasic (increases fire), not sattvic (calming), no matter how purely vegetarian it might be. That same tempeh burger, frozen, will be somewhat deadening (tamasic) because of the way it has been processed.

THE GUNAS IN FOOD: *Food affects the mind and body*

Sattvic food:

promotes calm clear mind, builds strong tissues and ojas. Supports a light clear approach to life. In excess, some experience it as ungrounding. Examples: most fresh easy-to-digest vegetarian food, both cooked and raw, including fresh milk, grains, legumes, steamed veggies, fresh fruits, ghee. Sattvic food is made with love.

THE GUNAS IN FOOD (Cont'd)

Rajasic food:

supports fiery assertive mind and physical endurance. It is often used when we are working hard physically. In excess, it can create fermentation, with possible inflammation. Examples: avocados, chickpeas, garlic, chile. Caffeine (including coffee, black tea, chocolate). (Green tea has a milder effect.) Eggs, cheese. Fresh high-quality animal meats. Alcohol, drugs (initial effect). Fermented foods and foods that ferment. Freshly canned foods. Food made with fury, irritation, or a competitive edge.

Tamasic food:

promotes grounding and completion, as well as inertia or numbness. Dulls the mind in excess. Examples: Onions, mushrooms, meats. Leftovers. Processed or microwaved foods. Frozen foods. Alcohol, drugs (long-term effect). Food made with indifference or apathy. (4)

Positive example: roasted onions to help you ground, if not prohibited by your spiritual practice.

THE NOBLE POTATO:
ONE EXAMPLE OF HOW PREPARATION MATTERS

SATTVIC:	RAJASIC:	TAMASIC:
Baked potato	Fresh french-fried potatoes	Frozen French-fried potatoes
Steamed potatoes	Fried potatoes, like fresh home fries	Potatoes with lots of mushrooms and onions
Sauteed potatoes, in small amount of oil, low heat	Potato with garlic and chili	Potatoes and bacon
(Fresh potato juice?! If it is well-digested.)	Fresh potato salad with pickles, mayo and mustard	Potato salad that was made 2-3 days ago (old)

A TYPICAL DAY,
IF "TYPICAL" WAS REALLY POSSIBLE IN EATING:

A Sattvic Day:	A Rajasic Day:	A Tamasic Day:
Fresh fruit or a freshly made hot cereal, like rice, oatmeal, whole wheat	Eggs, with salsa or tomato sauce as an option Fresh bread	Frozen "veggie" sausage with a bread or muffin from the freezer, toasted
Fresh veggie soup Homemade muffins Fresh salad	Hummus Avocado salad Fresh bread	Canned soup Cheese Store-bought crackers or bread
Fresh fruit or nuts as a snack	Store-bought yogurt, with a very fresh date	Store-bought yogurt, close to its expiration date
Homemade pasta and sauce with all fresh, mild ingredients	Soft cheese quiche with garlic and plenty of spices	Fresh or frozen mushroom onion lasagna

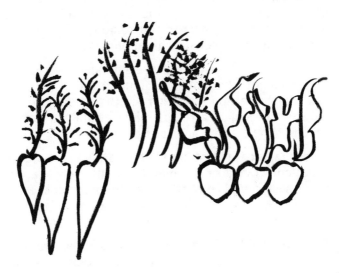

ASSESSING YOUR OWN
BALANCE OF THE GUNAS IN FOOD

It is easy enough to assess for yourself your guna balance in the intake of food. Write down everything you eat for three to five days (see FOOD DIARY which follows), hopefully recording it with as much love and a minimum of harsh judgments about yourself, whatever you are eating. Circle the sattvic (FRESH) foods, put an arrow on the rajasic (SPICY, FERMENTED) ones, underline the tamasic (PROCESSED, FROZEN, CANNED, ALCOHOL, DRUGS) items.

Note: Here in the U.S., I consider sugar to have either rajasic or tamasic effects. Eaten in moderation, it can give you a bit of a zip and possibly some fermentation, thereby it is rajasic. Eaten in excess, you can feel sedated and heavy, otherwise known as tamasic. Though if you've ever been to India, you know sugar is sattvic, because it's been made with love, blessed by the deities, and given as prasad at every ceremony, right? It's fair to note that sugar is used therapeutically in India by Ayurvedic physicians to calm certain illnesses or imbalances. My experience as a Western nutritionist in the U.S. is that we're usually better off without sugar, in the main.

In evaluating your current food style, look where the bulk of your choices lie. Are most of your foods sattvic, rajasic, or tamasic, or is there pretty much of a balance of two or more? Are you happy with the way you eat? If so, no need to go further. If you sense you could use food more effectively for healing, consider the following:

If you are dealing with depression, lethargy, fatigue, or excess weight, check out your tamasic food total. Is it high? You may be feeling low, then. Consider adding more fresh foods on a regular basis. You might even do an experiment: a week of fresh food, and see how you feel.

If your rajasic food total was hefty, are you feeling irritable, impatient, cranky, or inflamed (or do the people around you irrationally complain of this, even though you know you are perfect?) It's worth thinking about backing off on the spices or caffeine, perhaps.

Your sattvic total is virtuous, but you still feel crummy? Take a look at the discussion about prana, tejas and ojas. Your energy cushion may need some support.

FOOD DIARY:

DATE	WHAT I ATE:	TIME OF DAY:	PLACE:	HOW I FELT:
BREAK-FAST				
LUNCH				
DINNER				
SNACK				

SNEAKY SUBSTITUTIONS:

When we look at the mental qualities of sattva, rajas and tamas in our lives as a whole, we may see that we substitute the need for one of these in one part of our lives with that quality expressed in food, instead. Sneaky substitutions, these might be called. Let me explain further. For example, you might be needing to stay at home and rest, a reasonable tamasic urge to nest. If you ignore this urge and keep working hard outside your home, giving yourself little chance to rest, you may start compensating for your real need to rest by eating heavy, tamasic food, while you're out running around. These could be donuts, apple pie, enchiladas, burgers; heavy foods run the gamut. And yet your original need to rest goes unfulfilled. Here you're yearning for tamas in a particular area, your home, and yet instead you're giving it to yourself in another area, your food and stomach. Often these sneaky substitutions do not work and only leave us feeling cheated.

Other examples: you want to speak out about something you care about passionately, yet only go so far as to eat spicy foods (rajas). Or you may be yearning for more sattva in the form of quiet meditative time. Since you have not found a way to create more quiet retreat time, you find yourself choosing sattva instead in the form of an intensely focused vegetarian diet. You will be able to tell if you are on target in your expression of the gunas in your life if you feel basically satisfied. If you are feeling frustrated, ungrounded, or sluggish, something needs balance, and it is not always food. (To clarify here: I do not mean to imply that all spicy food urges should be met with speaking out, heavy foods with rest, or vegetarian diets with meditation. These are only three hypothetical examples out of many.)

It can be easy for us humans to pretend to be coming from the space of one guna, when we're really centered in another. A common one in my experience is working to hold with a sattvic neutral state of mind in the midst of conflict, only to erupt in rage later. For some of us, this rage is too scary, unacceptable, or impossible to express, and so we eat instead. Here we've gone from a rajasic state of anger masked as sattvic mellowness to dowsing the still unexpressed anger in a tamasic food eat-it-all out! Do you follow me?

POLARITY ENERGETIC NUTRITION:
FOOD AND THE ELEMENTS:

We have been looking at the gunas and food. This may be all you want to consider for now, and it is plenty. Stop right here and let yourself chew for a while. On the other hand, if you want to explore more, we look next at food and the elements.

Randolph Stone had a fine sense of the subtle energetics of food, and a deep appreciation for foods' relationship to nature as a whole. His way of approaching this was simple. Foods growing under the ground he considered earthy and building, like potatoes or carrots. Those close to the moist soil, growing close to the ground, he categorized as watery and cleansing, such as melons or squash. Those higher off the ground, which lie directly in the path of the sun's rays, are considered fiery and stimulating, such as beans, grains, or seeds like sunflowers. Foods growing in trees he considered airy and oxidizing, such as lemons or almonds. (5) Both gardeners and eaters can appreciate this common sense picture of the elements and its signature of "similars".

Stone also looked at the elements in terms of the state in which they manifested. As in Ayurveda, he associated earth with solid foods, water with liquid ones, fire with warm or spicy foods, and air with gaseous foods. He perceived that on a subtle level, the earthy (solid), watery (liquid), fiery (warm or spicy), and airy (gaseous) foods nourish not only the physical body, but the energetic currents as well. An excess of one food might over-stimulate one current or energetic zone compared to another, creating imbalance and subsequent problems. He maintained, *"Our constitution craves and attracts what we wish to build up or store in the body as essential elements or tissues..."* (6) *"Foods which contain more than one element in them serve those essences in our diet. Naturally, a balance must be maintained or the Polarity may be upset. Too much of any one stimulating food alone opposes the other factors and detracts from their share of energy currents in the body's economy."* (7)

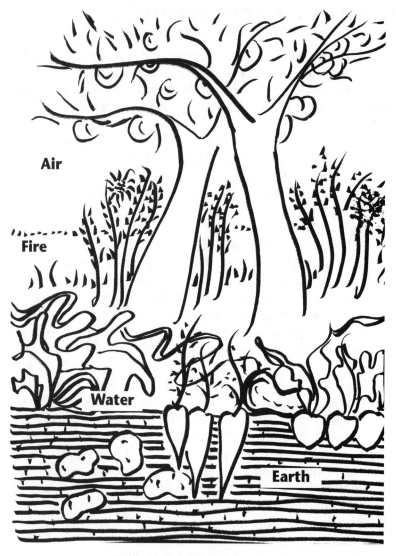

Food and the Elements

When we *are* craving something, it can feel far from "in balance". Yet it is interesting to explore our cravings a little further, in light of what they do for us. In one Polarity session I did with an insightful client, we began to explore her addiction to Pepsi. She was frustrated with the amount of weight she had put on, and was working hard to eliminate most sugar and sweets from her regime. Yet she just had to have a couple of Pepsi's every day. Starting out, it looked to both of us like the soft drink just added a sweet (=earthy), wet (=watery), heavy (=what earth and water both do for us) quality to her days, something she had in abundance already. Yet as I asked her to describe what it was about the drink that attracted her, her words revealed a different picture. She described it as "bubbly" "light" "a break" "forbidden". It had an airy quality for her, in its carbonation, that balanced the heavy grind of her current life. It tipped both of us off to which element needed to be invited into her life more, namely, the air.

ASSESSING YOUR OWN
BALANCE OF THE ELEMENTS IN FOOD

Like the gunas in food, you can pretty easily assess for yourself your elemental balance in the intake of food. Again, write down everything you eat for three to five days (or just pull out that first honest record), again recording it with as much love and a minimum of harsh judgments about yourself. When you're complete with your record, put a circle around all the roots (earth), draw a wavy line around the greens, melons, squash and other water foods, a star by the beans, grains, and seeds for fire, and a dotted line around the foods that grow in trees, the airy items. If something felt extra heavy, double-circle that. Liquids, add an additional wavy line to them. You can even get elegant and color code your choices, if you like. The point is, how does your balance of elements look? Are you eating mainly from one or two categories, or ideally, all of them?

Where do flesh foods lie in these categories? Dr. Stone never addressed this as he was strongly in favor of a vegetarian diet. My best estimate is: if you eat meat, poultry or eggs, you can consider these fiery and earthy, while fish is fiery and watery.

How do you evaluate yourself and use this as a tool for change? Say you are a hot-tempered person who tends to get headaches when under stress. You analyze your diet and see you're heavy on salsa, chips, refried beans, and tacos. Your only "green" in your diet is the lettuce in your tacos! Here it could be said you're feeding your fire too much. It might be time for more calming cooling greens, or some fresh fruit snacks, or simply more fresh water.

On the other hand, Dr. Stone generally advocated that a person of a given constitutional type was likely to need more of that same element in their diet. He would probably support you in sticking with your protein-rich regime of beans and grains (fiery foods for a fiery person), while urging you to expand your options, so that your other elemental energies could also be fed. He suggested, for example, that an earthy person would need more potatoes, and an airy soul, more lemons. Rather than give up all fiery foods, as Ayurveda might recommend, a Polarity Therapist might ask you to add in more earth, water, and air foods, and then see how you respond to that.

IN SUMMARY

Much of Dr. Stone's approach to food was simple and commonsensical. For readers familiar with the complex food rules of Ayurveda, Polarity's energetic nutrition can sound quite simple. And it is. Yet, it can also work quite well. Stone advocated simple meals, with a minimum of complicated food combining. He strongly urged that your food be well chewed. The biggest meal of the day was to be in the middle of the day, with supper being considerably lighter. Ever an advocate for the liver, he nixed any practices which could cause that organ to suffer, such as late night eating, over eating or excessive drinking, fried foods, and cooked oils.

Polarity looks first at the elements in foods, Ayurveda works with the elements in terms of how they manifest as tastes and textures. Polarity recommends eating some foods from each elemental group, with a primary focus on foods similar to your constitutional type. In Ayurveda, the intention is to get a blend of all six tastes (sweet, sour, salty, pungent, bitter, astringent) in any meal.

POLARITY
ENERGETIC NUTRITION: GROUNDED IN NATURE

Healing food choices are based on the elements.

POLARITY CONSTIT- UTIONAL TYPE:	CHOOSE MORE FOODS WITH THIS QUALITY:	EXAMPLES:
Air	Air	Foods that grow high above the ground, in trees: citrus, nuts, fruit. Also acid foods & fermented foods.
Fire	Fire	Foods that grow mid-height, catching much sunlight: grains, legumes, peas, seeds. Also: garlic, onions, ginger, chiles, spices.
Water	Water	Foods that grow close to the moist ground or in the water: leafy greens, melons, squash, cucumbers. Sea foods. Dr. Stone also included milk & dairy in this category.
Earth	Earth	Foods growing under the ground: roots of all kinds, including potato, carrot, beet. Also: sweets & starches & fats are included in this category.

"Our constitution craves and attracts what we wish to build up or store in the body as essential elements or tissues." (8)

AYURVEDIC NUTRITION: BASED ON THE ELEMENTS,
as they are perceived by the senses
and received by the doshas
as taste, texture, and other qualities.

Constitutional Type (dosha as prakruti)	Choose more foods with these tastes:	These textures:	Other supportive qualities:	Foods to use less frequently:
Vata (air-ether)	sweet, sour, salty	smooth, creamy, moist, oily, soft	warm	rough, dry, crispy, cold, frozen, pungent, bitter, astringent
Pitta (fire-water)	sweet, bitter, astringent	dry, rough, dense, fresh,crispy, hard	cool	oily, spicy hot, light, sour, salty, fermented
Kapha (earth-water)	pungent, bitter, astringent	dry, light, crispy, fresh, rough, clear	warm	oily, cold, heavy, sweet, salty, sour, dense

(9)

TASTE AND HEALING:

The taste of a food or herb is important in understanding its dynamic in healing. In Ayurveda, some tastes are used for cleansing (pungent, bitter and astringent); others for building (sweet, sour and salty). Dr. Stone also considered sweet taste building, and he used bitter taste to stimulate digestion. Foods for building tend to be pleasant tasting, while herbs for cleansing by their nature can taste quite bad. Both are needed in the scheme of things, in varying proportions.

Stone also used taste to support each constitutional type in their healing, although not in the exact same way an Ayurvedic physician would. Both systems agree that taste is a key to balancing health and digestion, yet sometimes they approach it in quite different ways. Rather than trying to defend one system or the other, I've presented both perspectives in the appendix: **KEY DIFFERENCES BETWEEN AYURVEDIC AND POLARITY NUTRITION.** You can see for yourself the similarities and differences in how each uses taste for healing.

TASTE TEST:

Taste can be used to gain perspectives on your needs. Here is a chance to explore for yourself which tastes are most appealing to you right now. Obviously, sweet taste can be a lot easier to love than a bitter one, yet sometimes it is surprising what our bodies crave for their healing.

Get together six of the following ingredients, one from each category:

SWEET: banana, raisins, or grape
SOUR: lemon, pickle, or umeboshi plum
SALTY: a pinch of mineral salt, black salt, or seaweed
PUNGENT: a little bit of chile, salsa, or black pepper
BITTER: a small amount of fresh raw chopped dandelion greens or other leafy green, bay leaf, or a drop of grapefruit seed extract
ASTRINGENT: a pinch of triphala (the Ayurvedic colon tonifying herbal combination), a witch hazel leaf or drop of witch hazel extract, a persimmon, or a very unripe banana

If you choose to do this with friends, you can arrange enough of each taste for everyone on its own plate, close your eyes and pass them around. Take a small bite of each taste. Which attract you? Do any repel you? It's good to have some water on hand in case you hit something that does not appeal at all.

TASTE TEST (Cont'd)

From a classical Ayurvedic perspective, taste can be an indicator of which doshas need balance. If you find sweet, bitter, and astringent tastes most appealing, your pitta dosha probably is yearning for balance. While sweet, sour, and salty being most attractive tips you off to the need to tend to vata. Yet what sane Kapha is going to go exclusively for bitter, pungent, and astringent?! Often we are not so neat and tidy as this in our cravings. Yet, if you find yourself really enjoying the bitter flavor, for example, your body is likely to be letting you know it would appreciate some cleansing. To get a further Polarity perspective on taste, see the appendix, **KEY DIFFERENCES.**

ABOUT CHOICE:

In this chapter four major variables have been introduced in terms of nourishment: ourselves with our individual needs and habits, the gunas (qualities) in food, the elements in food, and the tastes of foods. I've also suggested that we cannot create a nourishment plan without considering ourselves in the context of our families and communities. This is a lot to juggle. And yet, if you are ready, I'd like to invite you to open to one final variable in nourishment: choice.

In our country at this time, we are fortunate to be able to choose, most of us, how we will eat and what we will eat, as adults. This means if we want to eat more fresh foods, usually we can (though Alaskans and Montanans may not have the same variety Californians currently have.) If we decide we want to eat earthier root foods like carrots, we're likely to be able to do this. Or if we decide to eat less sweets and more bitter greens, it is a choice we can make. This means if we decide we want to try a sattvic purifying diet for three or four days, we're likely to be able to do it, at least in terms of being able to obtain the food and pursue our choices.

However, there are common conditions, such as childhood, where such freedom to choose your own food is not so present. If I were to say, " I am 46 and I live in Santa Fe, New Mexico", I'm talking about two variables, my age and where I live. One is a matter of choice (my home location) and the other is not (my age). We're constantly moving back and forth between conditions where we have a choice, and conditions which are apparently just given. (Like my age: I can accept it gratefully or gracefully, or resist it; it's still my age.) As children, our ages affected deeply how much say we had about what we ate. For most of us, we could accept what we were fed graciously, gratefully, passively, or with deep resistance, yet in most cases we weren't able to break out of what was offered on the table and feed ourselves whatever we wanted. Similar examples can crop up while traveling or visiting someone else's home for an extended period.

Patterns build up after years of little choice in childhood. It is important to wake up to the fact that (hopefully) now we're in a different situation, with more choices available. This in itself can be bewildering, so many choices after so few. Right now I'm just inviting you to notice the possibility that *you may have more choices than you realize.* This can be quite liberating, in and of itself.

If confusion arises with freedom, one simple way to address it is to consider the original questions which began this chapter, about digestion and what suits you. They are printed again here at the close of this chapter for your convenience.

If you are inclined, you can look at which of the gunas you want to be supporting now, and choose foods accordingly. Just work with one of these. Do you want to eat more fresh food (sattva), spicy stimulating food (rajas) or heavier grounding food (tamas)? That is enough as a starting point.

Or, you can ask yourself what your current focus is: cleansing, building, or maintaining. There is more information about specific foods for each of these processes in the following chapters.

MENTAL CHOICES, PHYSICAL CHOICES:

There are choices our minds make and choices our bodies make, and I'd like to make a distinction between these. We're grown up (presumably), we can eat what we want, and we do. Yet the mind and body don't always see food in the same way. Sometimes the mind has one idea, and the body has a very different one. The mind is often more idealistic than the body.

An experience I had many years ago comes to mind, when I was a fledgling nutritionist. My client was young and healthy and pregnant. She was determined to feed the baby inside her as purely as possible. In her mind at that time, that meant an organic vegan diet of fresh fruits, vegetables, grains, and beans. And yet she was beginning to have dizzy spells, and once she'd even passed out, as she neared her third trimester of pregnancy. My approach at that time was to honor all of my clients' choices and help them gather as much information about their health as possible. With that aim, she and I did a visualization together in which I asked my client to imagine her ideal picnic. She was mortified to find herself imagining a great big cheese pizza! Her mind and her body had obviously different ideas about what was healthy. It was up to her to reconcile the differences. She decided she needed to accept her body's yearnings for foods like pizza, and liberated her food plan to include more protein and more calcium-rich foods, which her body appreciated. The dizziness stopped, and she gave birth to a healthy, beautiful baby.

How can we tell a mental choice from a physical one? Usually a mental choice will manifest as some kind of idea like "It would be good if I ate............" Physical choices usually show up through our senses and actions. A particular food may smell very good to us, our body wants it. Or we find ourselves eating something before we've even thought about it! One style of choice is not better than another, in my mind, they each have their wisdom, and both need to be taken into account in any nourishment plan. If your body adores ice cream sundaes and you've decided to forgo all sugar, your body's desire for sugar is unlikely to disappear simply because your mind has chosen not to eat it! Negotiations are often needed.

In the years I was in practice as a nutritionist, I often suggested negotiation to my clients as a way to work with their bodies on these issues. Often our body is willing to trade one pleasure for another, although not always. Perhaps it is willing to trade sugar for bubble baths, or regular weekly Polarity sessions, or a walk in the woods. Cutting something out and simultaneously adding in something else that is satisfying can strongly increase the probability that your designed nourishment plan will succeed. It takes skill, patience, and flexibility to sort these differences out for ourselves. It's okay to take as much time as you need. If you are interested in pursuing this mind-body relationship further, there's more about this in chapter 8.

CHAPTER SYNOPSIS:

NOURISHMENT:

Is what I eat easily digestible for me?

Does it support my health and well-being?

Does it help create a calm, grounded center inside me?

Is it ethical, from my perspective?

If I were to change anything in the way I eat or drink now to meet my needs more effectively, what would it be?

RESOURCES IN NOURISHMENT:

Ballentine, Rudolph, *Diet & Nutrition: A holistic approach*, even-handed, understandable coverage of both Western and Ayurvedic nutrition.

Burger, Bruce, *Esoteric Anatomy: The Body as Consciousness*, see p. 345-353 for a well-organized discussion of Polarity nutrition.

Champion, James, RPP, HoloChromatic Life Sciences, PO Box 159, Nellysford, VA, 22958, phone: (888) 501-3273 or (804) 361-2042, email: mycolors@aol.com, has integrated Polarity Therapy, color, and the five elements in a unique and stimulating approach to nourishment.

Colbin, Annemarie, *Food and Healing*, coherent, clear, macrobiotic.

Colbin, Annemarie, *The Book of Whole Meals*, nice macrobiotic recipes, easy to follow, with a seasonal focus.

Davies, Stephen, and Alan Stewart, *Nutritional Medicine: The drug-free guide to better family health*, (an American version by Avon is currently out of print, regrettably). Best discussion of the specifics of therapeutic Western nutrition that I've seen.

Flaws, Bob, *The Book of Jook: Chinese Medicinal Porridges, A Healthy Alternative to the Typical Western Breakfast.* The Chinese equivalent of Ayurvedic kichadi, articulately written with a strong focus on healing.

Johari, Harish, *The Healing Cuisine: India's Art of Ayurvedic Cooking*, about the gunas: p. 64-68.

Jones, Marjorie Hurt, *The Allergy Self-Help Cookbook*, major allergy reference.

Joshi, Sunil V., *Ayurveda and Panchakarma: The Science of Healing and Rejuvenation*, good discussion about Ayurvedic nutrition: p. 129-156.

Lad, Usha and Vasant, *Ayurvedic Cooking for Self-Healing*, includes specific therapeutic uses of foods and tasty south Indian-style foods.

Madison, Deborah, *Vegetarian Cooking for Everyone*, grounded, accessible approach, yummy recipes.

Morningstar, Amadea, *Ayurvedic Cooking for Westerners*, focuses on the gunas and easy-to-prepare Western recipes, with recipes for Polarity Therapy as well.

Morningstar, Amadea and Urmila Desai, *The Ayurvedic Cookbook*, good coverage on the constitutional types with delicious west Indian-style recipes from Mataji Desai.

The Murrieta Foundation, *Murrieta Hot Springs Vegetarian Cookbook*, the book to go to for recipes and information about Polarity nutrition, with a wide range of classic American-style vegetarian fare, for Purifying, Health-Building, and Gourmet Vegetarian eating, including recipes from their famous Spa cuisine.

Potts, Phyllis, *Going Against the Grain: Wheat-Free Cookery*, Central Point Publishing, 21861 S. Central Point Road, Oregon City, OR 97045, 1992. Good American standards, without the wheat.

Reading, Chris M. and Ross S. Meillon, *Your Family Tree Connection: How to Use Your Past to Shape Your Future Health*, fascinating and readable paperback from this Australian psychiatrist, using medical family trees to sleuth out unrealized nutritional needs.

Stone, Randolph, *Health Building*, the original reference for Polarity Energetic Nutrition.

Stone, Randolph, *Polarity Therapy*, esp. vol. I, bk 3, p. 105-116, and vol II, p. 202-213.

Tiwari, Maya, *Ayurveda: A Life of Balance: The Complete Guide to Ayurvedic Nutrition & Body Types with Recipes*. In this soulful approach to Ayurveda, the author explores consciousness and food, and food preparation as spiritual practice, with many delicious, simple dishes along the way.

Wood, Rebecca, *The New Whole Foods Encyclopedia: A Comprehensive Resource for Healthy Eating*, integrates Western nutrition, Ayurveda, and traditional Chinese medicine in descriptions of common as well as rare foods. A lot you might want to know about food and healing.

VI.

CLEANSING

Understanding the Ayurvedic Concept of the Dhatus, the Seven Tissues, as They Relate to Cleansing and Health.

"We must dig deep and find the life energy and engage its attention and assist Nature's process of elimination, oxidation, circulation, liver function, bowel and kidney action, etc. Nature is grand, if we but understand."
STONE, *HEALTH BUILDING, P. 29*

Both Polarity and Ayurveda have unique perspectives on cleansing. The Ayurvedic concept of the *dhatus*, the seven levels of tissue health, offers help in both cleansing and building. I would like to go into this in greater detail in these next two chapters, because it puts both Ayurvedic practices and Dr. Stone's three Polarity food processes into perspective. It offers direct guidance on how often to do what, why, and when.

In Ayurveda, cleansing and building take into account the dhatus, the seven levels of tissue health. From an Ayurvedic view, after we eat our food, it moves into the digestive tract, and from there into the plasma. This is also the view of Western nutrition: nutrients are absorbed from the small intestine, primarily, into the bloodstream. This fluid plasma is the first tissue, called *rasa* in Sanskrit. Where Ayurvedic nutrition proceeds from here is different than Western nutrition, and it can be helpful when applied to Western nutrition as well as other systems for healing.

In Ayurveda, it is understood that nutrients spend about five days in each tissue, dependent on the strength of each tissue's digestive capacity. (1) Food is absorbed into the plasma (*rasa*), and after five days, whatever excess of nourishment is there proceeds into the next deeper level of tissue, the blood cells (*rakta*). After five days there, whatever is left is sent on to the muscle (*mamsa*) and so forth, until all seven levels of tissues have been nourished, ideally. We nourish successively plasma (*rasa*), blood cells (*rakta*), muscle (*mamsa*), fat (*meda*), bone (*asthi*), marrow and nerves (*majja*), and reproductive tissue (*artava* and *shukra*, female and male, respectively).

Digestion, the Dhatus (Tissues) and Ojas

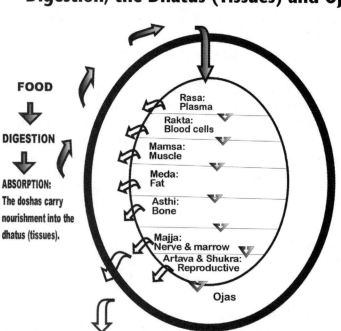

ELIMINATION: The doshas carry wastes (malas) out of each tissue. If toxic waste is not carried away and released, it can build up as ama (accumulated toxic waste) in the tissues and the GI tract, impairing absorption and healthy tissue metabolism.

CLEANSING: occurs at each tissue level as waste is carried away from each tissue by the doshas.

BUILDING AND REJUVENATION: occurs as each tissue increases in health and vitality. Ojas, our vital energy cushion, is built from the excess energy remaining after each tissue has been nourished.

NOURISHMENT OF THE DHATUS (TISSUES)

TISSUE (DHATU):	NAME IN SANSKRIT:	WHEN THIS TISSUE IS FED, DAYS AFTER EATING:	FUNCTIONS OF THE DHATUS:
Plasma	*rasa*	0-5	nourishment
Blood cells	*rakta*	6-10	invigoration, circulation of prana
Muscle	*mamsa*	11-15	establishing form
Fat	*meda*	16-20	lubrication, love, production of hormones
Bone	*asthi*	21-25	structure, support
Marrow and nerves	*majja*	26-30	to fill bone
Reproductive			reproduction, creativity
Female	*artava*	31-35	
Male	*shukra*	31-35	

If we do a five day fast, we have helped cleanse the plasma, and these good effects will be shared to some extent with all the deeper tissues. If we carry out a sensible cleansing program for ten days, we have reached to the level of the blood cells, and so on. Congestion and waste in one tissue impairs the flow of nourishment to the deeper tissues, and cleansing that preliminary tissue helps. One simple example of congestion and waste in the plasma is arteriosclerosis, in which the plasma in our blood vessels is congested with excess fat, known as cholesterol.

Chronic conditions take a while for us to create. Likewise, it can take more than five days to see a difference in many conditions. Dr. Stone mentioned this fact repeatedly. From the Ayurvedic perspective, if we have developed a nerve disorder like multiple sclerosis or Parkinson's disease, this has probably happened over a length of time, even years. Stress, toxics, lack of proper rest, nourishment or exercise slowly deteriorate first one tissue then the next until the nervous tissue is no longer getting what it needs. Likewise, to cleanse and rebuild this tissue takes time and persistence. In this case, we are unlikely to see much difference in a healing program, even if it is an appropriate one for us, until we have stuck with it for a minimum of 30 days. (see NOURISHMENT OF THE DHATUS chart, *majja*)

The ancient process of cleansing in Ayurveda is called *Pancha Karma*, five actions (or processes of cleansing). This series starts with pre-procedures like steams and oil massage to soften us up and draw our wastes to the surface. It then goes on to the actual cleansings, which include nasal cleansing, enemas, purgation, and other processes (such as vomiting and blood letting). In the United States, most people participating in a Pancha Karma cleanse will do only some of these processes, usually the steams, massage, and nasal and colon cleansing. In a week to ten days, this is plenty to do. And it can be expected to offer a good cleansing to the first two levels of tissues, the plasma and blood cells. Traditionally, however, Pancha Karma was done for twenty-eight days or more. This gave all seven levels of tissue health time to clear and cleanse. And thirty-day programs of Pancha Karma are still available in some clinics in India. However, for most of us, it takes extraordinary effort to be able to come up with the time and money to be able to do such a cleansing retreat. Hence, the development of the shorter programs here.

When you are dealing with a serious condition, which reaches into the nerves or reproductive tissue, longer programs of cleansing and building will give you the greatest benefits. In Polarity as well, Stone often emphasized that in order to be able to see the benefit of specific foods, one had to apply them with concerted effort over time. Patience is a primary asset in these situations, something neither our upbringing as Westerners nor Western medicine itself has inclined us much to apply.

There are many implications to this theory of the dhatus. First, if we cleanse one tissue, it will help them all to some extent, because 1) waste obstructs the flow of nourishment within a tissue and from that tissue to other tissues, and 2) waste can penetrate from one tissue into deeper tissues. Cleaning out even one room in your house helps. Cleaning out all the rooms can feel really fantastic. However, it takes time and effort. So we do what we can.

The relatively new technique of dark field examination of the blood is a way that Western medicine examines the health of the first two tissue levels, rasa and rakta. The plasma and blood cells are clearly revealed in this microscopic technique. A traditional Ayurvedic physician would evaluate the health of these tissues, plus the other five dhatus, through pulse.

In both Polarity and Ayurveda, the focus is usually on cleansing first, then building. The reason for this, as explained in Ayurveda, is as follows. When toxic waste, *ama* as it is called in Sanskrit, builds up in any tissue, it is like garbage in a stream, literally. Imagine then, that rich nutrients are put into that stream. In a stream, clumps of algae begin to grow around the garbage, fed by nutrient-rich run-off. In the body, whether it is building foods or vitamin supplements, protein powders and the like, inevitably some of the building nutrients accumulate around the *ama*, toxic waste, causing it to grow. The *ama* itself can grab up and sequester nutrients, so that the nutrients don't get to the tissues that need them. The channel, the stream itself, can become blocked, causing further congestion. In the body these channels are called *srotas*, and the congestion can become a cause of subsequent disease, such as allergy. (2)

Another example could be taken from house painting. When you paint a wall, you need to wash it first. If you don't, the fresh paint will bubble up around the globs of dust and dirt, creating a very different effect from that which you intended.

Now there are times when you can be very weak AND very dirty. This is tough. In Ayurveda, a good Ayurvedic physician won't let you do Pancha Karma in this situation. And in Polarity, this is where Dr. Stone's health building diet can be extremely useful. It is easy on the organs, especially the liver, and will gently build you up until you are strong enough to cleanse. Or if you are working with Ayurveda instead, the *vaidya*, Ayurvedic physician, will recommend an appropriate program.

Because this is a chapter about cleansing, that is what is highlighted. It is not unusual to need building as well as cleansing. There is much information about how to rejuvenate in the following chapter.

POLARITY BASICS TO CONSIDER IN CLEANSING:

When planning for cleansing, it is important to remember the organs that will be most active as you cleanse. These include the colon, the kidneys, the skin, and the lungs. Respectively, they help you clear out solid wastes (earth element), fluids (water), perspiration and heavy metals (fire), and air. Each of the elements can act as a vehicle for carrying deeper wastes out of your system. Sweating, for example, is a great way to excrete mercury from the body. You want to support all these systems as you cleanse.

SUPPORTS IN CLEANSING:

Colon	Kidneys	Skin	Lungs	Brain & Nervous System
colonics or home enemas or bastis (Ayurvedic enemas)	alkalizing diet enough pure water	salt glow dry brush massage	deep breathing Polarity body work	rest 5-pointed star: Polarity body work
laxatives	rest	showers	pranayama	relax, don't work so much!

Food is kept simple, including simple food combinations, to give the entire digestive system rest. In Polarity, an alkalizing, purifying diet is eaten. Information on both Polarity and Ayurvedic purifying processes follows.

AYURVEDA: CLEANSING THE TISSUES:

In Ayurveda, one always attends to the doshas and digestion first, then considers the metabolism of the dhatus, the deeper tissues. The thought is, if these major players, Vata, Pitta, and Kapha, are out of balance or the digestion is poor, little can be done for the dhatus until these issues have been corrected. If your car has suddenly stopped running, you would usually first check the function of the engine, rather than rush off to fix the bent fender. The dhatus are fed by healthy digestion, and this nutriment is delivered by the doshas. It has been said, "Diseases get automatically alleviated when the dhatus are brought to their normal state." (3) So information will be shared here about cleansing and building these tissues further, mainly for the reader with prior experience in Ayurveda. If you have a beginning interest in Ayurveda, remember that getting your digestion working well and your doshas in balance are the first priorities in addressing any physical challenges. Establishing a working relationship with an Ayurvedic physician can help you skillfully cleanse or build the deeper tissues without having to juggle all the details of specific food choices yourself.

There is a traditional assessment Ayurvedic practitioners do before recommending either cleansing or rejuvenation. They note:
1) the client's doshas: how are they doing?
2) any herbs or medicines being taken by their client
3) where the person lives, what is their normal environment and climate like? (Singapore is quite different in its effects from Montana, for example.)
4) the season: is it hot, cold, wet, dry? How might this be affecting the individual and their condition?

5) the physical strength of the person, including their digestive strength
6) their build and muscle tone
7) the strength of the dhatus
8) their client's diet, including when they eat foods and the tastes they prefer
9) their mental and emotional temperament (the gunas)
10) their constitution
11) their age. (4)

Usually if a person were to do Pancha Karma, they would eat a simple mono-diet of kichadi throughout the program. Kichadi is a mildly spiced one-pot meal of well-cooked mung beans, rice, and often, though not always, vegetables. The intention is to nourish and cleanse, while taking a load off the digestive tract. This simplification of food works remarkably well for many individuals. (5)

A core tenet of Ayurveda is: food must be digested well in order to have a balancing effect on the doshas and the dhatus. This means that the body digests it well, not just that our mind thinks it is an assimilable possibility. If you do not digest beans well in general, it is worth trying at least one serving of kichadi before committing to eight days of eating it during Pancha Karma. Similarly, in other non-Ayurvedic cleansing regimes, raw foods are often the norm. Some people do very well on this kind of program, others do not. A start for yourself in evaluating any cleansing food regime is: can I digest this? You may need to try a day or two of it to find out, before committing to a longer period.

To understand Ayurveda's approach to cleansing and building deeper tissues, it is helpful to know that each of the seven tissues is watched over by a specific dosha (see next page).

CLEANSING PRACTICES FOR THE DHATUS

DHATU	SUPPORTING DOSHA	CLEANSING MEASURES
plasma (*rasa*)	Kapha	pranayama
blood cells (*rakta*)	Pitta	pranayama
muscle (*mamsa*)	Kapha	regular enjoyable exercise
fat (*meda*)	Kapha	sweats, saunas
bone (*asthi*)	Vata	basti (Ayurvedic enemas), seaweed wraps
nerve & marrow (*majja*)	Kapha	aromatherapy
reproductive: female (*artava*)	Kapha	respect, devotional practices
male (*shukra*)	Kapha	respect, devotional practices

Pancha Karma is useful for cleansing all of the dhatus. Food and lifestyle regimes calming to a particular dosha will also help the specific dhatu(s) that it supports. Specific foods are sometimes recommended for cleansing specific dhatus; it is important to realize that these recommendations are based on supporting the dosha in charge of that dhatu. So for five of the seven dhatus (plasma, muscle, fat, nerve and marrow, and reproductive tissue) one focuses on cleansing Kapha, because Kapha watches over these dhatus. In cleansing blood cells, one focuses on Pitta and its balance; and for bone, Vata. This makes for unexpected and yet effective Ayurvedic recommendations. For example, Ayurveda approaches bone health in a different way than we normally would in the West. Vata rules the bones. To maintain strong bones, Ayurveda first makes sure the bone tissue is clear of impurities, by cleansing the colon, the seat of Vata, with gentle enemas if needed. Oil massage is used to support Vata and strengthen bone and muscle. Regular weight-bearing exercise and rest are other components of Ayurvedic bone support. If you are interested in further information related to Ayurvedic cleansing, see the RESOURCES section at the end of this chapter.

In the charts that follow, specific foods and herbs are suggested to cleanse each tissue. These are not comprehensive, just some of the more effective aids to get you started. Organic, unadulterated food is always recommended as a top priority for use with both cleansing and building. In Ayurveda, kichadi is considered the all-purpose tri-doshic cleanser for all dhatus, in conjunction with Pancha Karma. There are many good references about dosha-calming diets now. See particularly Lad, Tiwari, Johari, Morningstar, and Morningstar and Desai in the RESOURCES section.

Ayurveda: Cleansing the Tissues

Cleansing foods & practices

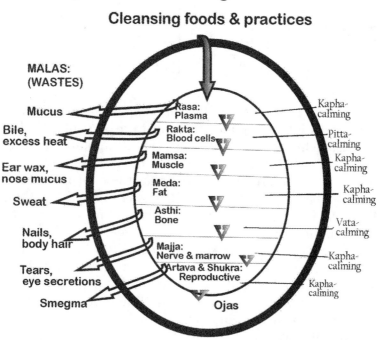

CLEANSING: occurs at each tissue level as specific waste is carried away from each tissue (dhatu) by the doshas. The primary wastes, urine and feces, are processed by the kidneys and digestive tract, and are also transported by the doshas. For optimal cleansing, one focuses on foods and practices calming to the dosha which watches over the specific tissue. So, for example, to cleanse the plasma, one would choose Kapha-calming foods.

AYURVEDA: CLEANSING FOODS FOR THE DHATUS

DHATU	CLEANSING FOODS FOR EACH DHATU
plasma (*rasa*)	Freshly made organic fruit and vegetable juices, especially those calming to Kapha, apples, oranges, carrots, artichokes, summer squashes, fresh greens, cumin-coriander-fennel tea, Polaritea, cleansing bitters
blood cells (*rakta*)	Fresh fruits and vegetables calming to Pitta, including cilantro, mint, pomegranate, fresh wheatgrass juice, barley greens, artichokes, string beans, summer squashes, asparagus, cucumber, mung bean sprouts, cleansing bitters
muscle (*mamsa*)	Fresh vegetables and fruits calming to Kapha, such as cabbage family, string beans, asparagus, artichokes, apples, turmeric tea, Polaritea, cleansing bitters
fat (*meda*)	All of the above, plus eliminating chemicals & adulterated fats from the diet; fresh greens including lettuce, watercress, parsley, broccoli; lemon, grapefruit with seeds, berries, pure fluids, cleansing bitters, pungent foods
bone (*asthi*)	Pure seaweeds, fresh juices calming to Vata including grape, papaya, lemon, eliminating sources of toxic metals from the diet, including cooking in aluminum; mantra
nerve & marrow (*majja*)	Avoiding foods with a build-up of toxic metals, plastics, & other neurotoxins; fresh cilantro, parsley, & celery may be of assistance. Much of the cleansing can also be more subtle here, as in how we nourish our minds and hearts: mantra, positive support, gratitude
reproductive: female (*artava*)	Eliminate hormones and hormone-stimulators from the diet, reduce animal fats (rich in chemotoxins), use fresh vegetables calming to Kapha, such as asparagus and watercress
male (*shukra*)	Similar to artava above in the clearing out of hormonal contaminants; asparagus is particularly clearing to the dhatu as a food

Note: There are many other cleansing tea options, see HERBS TO CLEANSE THE DHATUS chart which follows

HERBS TO CLEANSE THE DHATUS:

DHATU	sattvic herbs	rajasic herbs	tamasic herbs
RASA (PLASMA)	aloe vera* bayberry bibhitaki* burdock calamus dandelion pomegranate root bark (worms) red clover sage sarsaparilla wild cherry bark hibiscus (a little rajasic)	ajwan barberry cloves echinacea gentian goldenseal horsetail juniper berry mint mullein prickly ash (candida, worms) pennyroyal C turmeric rhubarb C senna C yarrow yellow dock	asafoetida/ hing valerian
RAKTA (BLOOD CELLS)	aloe vera* bayberry burdock juniper berry mint *myrrh** red clover sage wild cherry bark	barberry echinacea gentian bitters in general goldenseal horsetail mugwort mullein pennyroyal C turmeric yarrow yellow dock	asafoetida/ hing valerian
MAMSA (MUSCLE) includes organs	aloe vera* bibhitaki calamus dandelion (liver) juniper berry wild cherry bark (lungs)	barberry (liver) gentian (GI) hibiscus (heart) mugwort pennyroyal (uterus) C turmeric yarrow	asafoetida/ hing valerian
MEDA (FAT)	aloe vera* calamus fennel seed juniper berry	barberry (combine with turmeric) gentian horsetail rhubarb C turmeric	

HERBS TO CLEANSE THE DHATUS (Cont.):

DHATU	sattvic herbs	rajasic herbs	tamasic herbs
ASTHI (BONE)	aloe vera bibhitaki* guggul juniper berry myrrh *nirgundi* sarsaparilla	horsetail turmeric	asafoetida/hing valerian
MAJJA (NERVE MARROW)	aloe vera* *aromatherapy* bayberry, calamus juniper berry sage sarsaparilla wild cherry bark	ajwan hibiscus mugwort mullein turmeric	asafoetida/hing valerian
ARTAVA (FEMALE REPRO-DUCTIVE)	*aloe vera** calamus myrrh* sarsaparilla	hibiscus turmeric	
SHUKRA (MALE REPRO-DUCTIVE)	*aloe vera** calamus sarsaparilla	turmeric	

KEY:

* = also rejuvenative
herbs in italics = especially useful
C = caution, not for use in pregnancy. Other herbs may also fall into this category; double check with your healthcare practitioner for complete lists if you are pregnant or wanting to conceive.

Note: many herbs (not included here) work primarily to cleanse the digestive tract, which is the first place to begin cleansing. See *The Yoga of Herbs*, Lad and Frawley for more information about these. Any of these herbs, because of their tastes and qualities, could increase Vata dosha if used in excess. Much of the information presented here is compiled from The *Yoga of Herbs*, with appreciation especially to Dr. Frawley for his guidance. Any errors are my own.

STIMULATING DIGESTIVE FIRE IN THE DHATUS:

Each of the dhatus has its own digestive metabolism, hence certain herbs are used to strengthen the specific digestive fire of a dhatu needing cleansing, to burn up its ama, waste. This is an area that takes skill, and a good deal of experience to address well in Ayurveda. Poorly applied, herbs to strengthen digestive fire can increase Pitta, fire dosha, and possible inflammation. One relatively safe example of an Ayurvedic substance that is used for cleansing that is also fairly readily available is guggul. Guggul increases digestive fire in fat (*meda*) tissue. Often in the case of weight accumulation, the digestive fire in our fat tissue is low, and guggul can help reverse this condition. In general, eating pure food that suits you and that you respect, will also help tonify this digestive fire.

THE POLARITY PURIFYING PROCESS:

What I noticed often in my first years of teaching Energetic (Polarity) Nutrition, was that many of us Americans are uncomfortable with the idea of fasting. Now a few of us get so enamored of purifying, that we purify ourselves into the ground. Yet most of us sit around with the clutter accumulating inside the house we know as our body, and are reluctant to let a bit of it go. Consequently, an abundance of good information in Dr. Stone's books about cleansing goes largely untried. We are concerned that we will be weak, we will make ourselves sick, we will be unable to complete the fast, it is too radical, and so forth. All of these things are possible. And yet done properly for short periods of time, dire results are unlikely. And positive effects can be downright surprising, not to mention gratifying.

In my own experience, trying out Dr. Stone's suggestions has taught me much that I could have learned no other way. So when I am training professional Polarity Therapy students about Stone's three diet processes, my recommendation is to try at least one week of health-building diet and three days of purifying food processes. The feedback I get is that this is very helpful. It helps us understand directly what a difference a clear colon makes, and how much happier a sluggish liver is without cooked oil. And yet each person is different, and how much one person needs to cleanse can be very different than another.

ACID-ALKALINE BALANCE:

An alkalizing diet is used in purifying, to promote the most cleansing from the tissues. (See ENERGETIC NUTRI-TION: ACID-ALKALINE BALANCE chart which follows.) When the body becomes overly acidic, parasites, bacteria, fungus, viruses, even cancer can become more easily established. Shifting the internal pH of the body tissues in a more alkaline direction actively discourages the growth of these organisms and disease in our systems. One of the chief advantages of a well-designed vegetarian diet is that it is readily alkalizing, thereby warding off illness.

Simply, an alkaline diet contains foods that the body burns up in digestion into an alkaline ash. This occurs because the proportion of minerals in the specific foods are more alkaline. Alkaline-forming foods tend to be cleansing, especially to the kidneys. Most fresh fruits and vegetables, with the exception of prunes, plums and cranberries, are strongly alkalizing.

Acid-forming foods are generally building to the whole body, although not invariably. Acid-forming foods include all those foods that are metabolized to an acidic ash, once they've been thoroughly digested. These include most proteins, starches, and sweets, as well as the aforementioned prunes, plums, and cranberries. The less of these foods included in a purifying fast, the more intensely cleansing it will be. However, acid-forming foods, such as sprouted legumes or grains, also offer the bulk of calories and grounding influences. If you eliminate these entirely, depending on your constitution and blood-sugar balance, you may do fine or you may flounder mightily.

A potentially confusing point is that both alkaline-form-ing and acid-forming foods often do not <u>taste</u> the way they are ultimately metabolized. That is, a lemon, although it is sour and acid tasting in the mouth, is digested in the body into an alkalizing ash, making it a great cleanser. In general, fresh fruits and vegetables are strongly alkalizing, even those with sour taste. Dr. Stone investigated fairly thor-oughly in an experiential way the effects of alkalizing foods. Some of the results of his experiments with specific disorders are distilled in the CLEANSING HOME REMEDIES table, which concludes this chapter.

While alkalizing foods are highly valued for their cleans-ing function, occasionally even in illness we can become too alkaline. For example, in bladder irritation or infection, it is important to test the pH of the urine. If it is too acidic (that is, a pH of 6 or below), foods like carrot juice, vegeta-bles, and fruits other than plums and cranberries are used to rebalance. Yet if the urine is reading quite alkaline (pH 8 or above), the individual needs acid-forming substances, like cranberry juice or vitamin C. Otherwise, the tissues may become more irritated.

Stressful emotions are also potentially acidifying, as they catalyze the release of hormones which acidify the tissues. Polarity Therapist Farida Sharan has observed aptly how different emotions affect our acid-alkaline balance. Laughter, joy, love, and good company are alkalizing, as are rest, sleep, fresh air, and a moderate amount of exercise. Stress (and the hormones released by stress) acidify, as do fear, worry, anxiety, and anger. (6)

: *LIVER FLUSH:*

a blender:

e, apple, or grapefruit juice
on juice
ssed olive or almond oil
er root, peeled and chopped
(optional)
(optional, use with caution)

ollows closely one given in *Murrieta Hot Springs kbook*. The variations on ingredients and the
ynamics are my own.

tely with a cup or two of Polaritea:

er

root, coarsely chopped
eds
k seeds
ce root

her all ingredients over low heat for 10-15 min-
f heat and steep 30 minutes or more.

mall handful fresh peppermint

10 minutes or so, strain, and drink.

ENERGETIC NUTRITION: ACID-ALKALINE BALANCE
KEY: foods in italics=on the Purifying Diet

LIQUIDS:	*Blood purifying herb teas, such as dandelion root, nettle, red clover, burdock, turmeric, or triphala*	MOST CLEANSING
	Vitality Drink: Liver Flush	
↑	*Polaritea*	MOST
	Fresh wheat grass juice	ALKALINE
	Barley green, other young grass drinks	FORMING
	Fresh vegetable juices, fresh fruit juices	
	Pure water	
	Clear vegetable broths	
	Spirulina, chlorella, or wild blue green algae drinks (in moderation.) *	
	Unpasteurized apple cider vinegar *	
RAW FOODS: ↑	*Fresh fruits and vegetables*	
	Easily digestible raw sprouted seeds, grains, beans, esp. alfalfa, mung	
	Freshly made vegetable pickles, raw cabbage sauerkraut (homemade, free of sugar & chemicals)	ALKALINE-FORMING
COOKED FOODS:	*Steamed leafy vegetables*	
	Steamed root vegetables	
↓	*Cooked fresh fruits*	MILDLY
	Cooked sprouted grains, seeds & beans, esp. millet and mung	ACID-FORMING,
	Soaked dried fruits (except prunes & cranberries)	BUILDING
	Grains	
	Legumes, mung is esp. cleansing	
MINIMIZE IN FASTING, BETTER FOR BUILDING:	*Soaked almonds (up to 8 per day on purifying)*	
	Raw honey (small amounts)	
	Essene bread (if fresh)	
	Cold-pressed olive or flax oils, other oils	
	Avoid corn oil (thyroid inhibitor)	
	Ghee (heated fat)	
	Potatoes, cranberries, plums, prunes	
↓	Raw goat milk	
NOT FOR FASTING, DESIGNED FOR BUILDING OR GOURMET VEGETARIAN	Other raw nuts & seeds	
	Raw cheeses	
	Raw nut & seed butters	
	Nutritional yeast, vinegar, pickles	MORE
	Fish, poultry, eggs	BUILDING
	Cooked cheese & dairy, breads, tortillas, chapattis, roasted nut & seed butters, baked goods with oil or butter cooked into them	MOST ACID-FORMING

(7) This chart is loosely adapted with permission from Paul Pitchford, *Healing with Whole Foods*, revised edition, p. 240, for use with Polarity diets, with appreciation to him.

*=in excess, the high protein blue-green algae and green algae can be acidifying

So how might you do a purifying day? Let's look at it.

A TYPICAL PURIFYING DAY: Wake up, stretch.

* Drink a glass of LIVER FLUSH (see following pages)
* Follow immediately with 1–2 cups of POLARITEA
  (see following pages)

* Take a shower with salt glow (chapter 1)

* Wait at least two hours after the flush, or until you are
  thoroughly hungry, before choosing from the following
  foods to eat. You can prepare regular meals with these,
  or graze your way through purifying.

ALKALIZING FOOD FOR PURIFYING:

Fresh Fruits

apples	pear	
apricots	persimmon	
berries of all kinds	pineapple	
cantaloupe	pomegranate	
cherries	quince	
figs	strawberries	
grapes	tangerine	
grapefruit	watermelon	
honeydew		
kiwi	*Oils*	
kumquat	cold-pressed	
lemon	flax oil	
lime	extra-virgin	
mango	olive oil	
melons of all kinds	cold-pressed	
nectarine	sesame oil	
orange		
pawpaw		
peach		

Sweeteners

(keep to a
minimum)
soaked dried
fruits
raw honey

"Extras"

spirulina or blue
green algae, in
moderation
powered young
greens, like
Green Magma
or wheat grass
juice,
if well-tolerated

ORGANIC PREFERRED,
whenever possible

ALKALIZING FOOD FOR P

Fresh Vegetables

acorn squash	jicama
artichoke	kale
arugula	kohlrał
asparagus	lettuce
beans, snap	mache
bean sprouts	mizun:
beets	mustar
broccoli	okra
Brussels sprouts	onions
burdock root	pac ch
butternut squash	parsle
cabbage, all kinds	parsni
carrots	peas
celery	peppe
celtuce	pursla
chicory	radicc
collards	rutabá
cucumber	shallot
daikon radish	snow
dandelion greens	spagh
& root	spina
endive	sprou
escarole	squas
fennel	toma
fenugreek sprouts	turnij
and greens	zucch
garlic	
green beans	
greens of all kinds	
Jerusalem artichoke	

*Eat as often as you are hu
  as you like
* Breathe deeply.   * Rest.
* If you can, get some Pola
* End of the day: Rest, go t

VITALITY

Combine v

6 oz. fresh
1 Tbsp. fre
1 Tbsp. co
1 inch fresk
1–2 cloves
cayenne to

(8) This rec
Vegetarian
explanation

Follow imm

POLARITEA

Bring to a b
4 cups pure

Add:
1/2" fresh gi
1 Tbsp. fenne
1 Tbsp. fenug
1 1/2 tsps. lic
1 Tbsp. flax s

Cover and si
utes, or turn

Add:
1 Tbsp. dry o

Steep anothe

DYNAMICS, LIVER FLUSH

fresh fruit juice: alkalizing
fresh lemon: strongly alkalizing
olive oil: stimulates discharge of bile from liver
almond oil: more calming if there is inflammation, such as colitis
ginger root: stimulates digestion and circulation
garlic: rich in sulfur, detoxifying to liver
cayenne: cuts mucus

DYNAMICS, POLARITEA

ginger: warming, anti-oxidant, stimulates digestive fire
fennel: neutral energetic, clears gas, supports digestion & weight loss
fenugreek seeds: warming, strengthens digestive fire, builds tissues
licorice root: cooling, anti-inflammatory, soothing, laxative, brings out the best qualities of the rest of the spices, holds fluids in the body
flax seeds: laxative, builds immunity and ojas, helps membranes transmit a healthy charge from one part of the body to another
peppermint: cooling, digestive

These are the distilled modern recipes that are often used for Polarity Purifying. And yet it is interesting to look at Dr. Stone's original prescriptions, which follow:

ORIGINAL VERSIONS OF DR. STONE'S LIVER FLUSH:

TAKE ONE:
1–3 Tbsps. of pure, cold-pressed almond or olive oil
3–9 Tbsps. of fresh lime or lemon juice.

Stir together, drink. Follow with:

2 cups hot water with juice of 1/2 to 1 lemon in each cup.
(9)

TAKE TWO:
1–3 Tbsps. of pure, cold-pressed almond or olive oil
1 cup FRESH orange, grapefruit, pomegranate, or pineapple juice.
Follow again with the two cups of lemon water
described above.
(10)

TAKE THREE:
3–4 Tbsps. of pure, cold-pressed almond, olive or sesame oil
6-8 Tbsps. of fresh lemon juice (about a cup)
Add:
fresh ginger juice to taste.
"If you can get grapefruit, add the juice of one grapefruit or several oranges, and drink it."
"Chew and swallow three to six small cloves of garlic with the oil mixture. Then have the hot tea mentioned above without sweetening."
(11)

ONE ORIGINAL VERSION OF STONE'S POLARITEA:

Take two or more cupfuls of hot herb tea made of:
Licorice Root
Himalayan Mountain Violet
Anise or Fennel
Peppermint
Fenugreek

At the time of serving add:
fresh lemon juice
fresh ginger juice to taste
honey if desired ("Do not use honey with the liver flush.")

If constipated, use more licorice root and fresh garlic.

If experiencing diarrhea, use no licorice, ginger, or liver flush. Instead, use cinnamon sticks in the herb tea. Blackberry juice is also useful here. (12)

ABOUT THE LIVER FLUSH:

In recent years I find some younger students in need of more care for their livers, especially those dealing with higher levels of toxins concurrent with compromised livers. In this situation, the regular liver flush may stimulate queasiness or nausea. If this is the case, instead of the liver flush, begin by substituting the juice of half a lemon in a cup of pure warm water on rising instead. If even this stirs nausea uncomfortably, try plain hot water on rising for a week or more, up to a month. If this is well-tolerated, the lemon in hot water can be tried again. If this sits well over a one to two week period of daily use, a mild liver flush such as the Vitality Drink recipe given here, can be tried again. Fresh air, exercise, and reducing dramatically the intake of chemicals, intoxicants, recreational drugs, and stressful emotional conditions helps tremendously in these situations.

CLEANSING SUPPORTS:

Checking your own tongue is an easy Ayurvedic way to assess the relative need of your gut for cleansing. If there is a thick coat throughout the tongue, ama (waste) has accumulated throughout the gastro-intestinal tract. If there is a coat toward the back of the tongue, the waste has primarily gathered in the colon, the large intestine. Usually the coat will be white. If it has a yellowish hue, the liver is also in need of support and cleansing. As you follow a cleansing diet, whether Purifying or Health-Building, relative to your needs and past food choices, you can watch the changes on your tongue. Often more waste will accumulate for a few days, as it is being released into the digestive tract. This can be reflected by an even thicker coat on your tongue. Then, as the waste breaks down and is eliminated through your colon, your tongue will start to clear up. You can help this process along by gently scraping the coat off with a spoon or tongue scraper.

Fifty years ago, Dr. Stone recommended a colon cleanse which could be done at home in the bathroom simply by flushing shower water up the rectum. Today, what city water would be pure enough to be able to do such a technique safely? And yet one can do enemas with purified water, bastis (Ayurvedic enemas) with herbal teas or oils, or various laxatives or colon cleanses. Standard dosages are about one tablespoon of herb per cup of boiled water, then strained very well. For example, in Ayurveda, one tablespoon of triphala per cup of pure water is steeped, then put through a cheese cloth folded about eight times or so in a tea strainer. You want to get any powder or leaf residue out of the enema preparation, or it can clog up your application bag at some very inopportune moment. Temperature is also important, comfortable to the skin being best; teas cool down quickly.

In terms of perspiration and the skin, Dr. Stone's salt glow (chapter 1) is an excellent cleanser during a fast. Simply showering is helpful, because as we release toxins through the skin, they need to be washed away. Otherwise, we may simply reabsorb them.

Again, in cleansing the air element, it is important to give ourselves chances for deep breathing in fresh air during our cleanse.

It is important to consider how you will create a respite for your nervous system and mind as well as your body during this fast, as they usually get much stimulation in this world. These systems run on glucose, about 60 grams minimum of this simple carbohydrate each day. To minimize uncomfortable sensations, like headache, weakness, or nausea related to low-blood sugar, you want to give yourself enough glucose for the nervous system and brain to function happily. Some of us have abundant fat supplies that in this sort of situation can be converted into glucose for fuel. Some of us don't. For those in the second category, water fasts can be overly heroic ventures. Sixty grams of carbohydrate is equivalent to 240 calories, or about 2 1/2 apples, 1 1/2 oranges, a cup of carrot juice, or 6 cups of steamed kale. Remember to feed yourself as you fast.

If your adrenal glands are exhausted, in most cases you will need to build before you can consider cleansing.

THE CURRENTS AS CLEANSING SUPPORTS:

Polarity bodywork, Polarity chi gung and Polarity yoga (see chapter 2) all activate the flow of the currents, enabling accumulated congestion to clear out. It is important to combine breath with these for maximum beneficial effects.

Working with the transverse current supports our nervous system and our ability to relax and take in breath. Supporting the spiral current strengthens our digestive fire and helps clear old waste out of the digestive tract. Balancing the long lines is a potent way to free long-held emotional patterns and equilibrate each of the five elements flowing within the long lines.

STARS WITHIN US:

Polarity offers additional support for the nervous system in two geometrical patterns of bodywork release. They are called the five-pointed star pattern and the six-pointed star pattern. The five-pointed star connects our shoulders, hips, and head. If we stand up with our legs shoulder-width apart and stretch our arms straight out at our sides, we can see this star pattern in ourselves, like a giant starfish, as we did in some of the movements in chapter 2. A tremendous amount of nervous tension can be stored in this pattern, in the pelvis, shoulders, and neck. Receiving a Polarity Therapy bodywork session can be quite supportive during a cleanse. We can also work the pattern ourselves, with one hand massaging and holding the neck while the other works around the hip. Then we can work shoulder to hip, opposite hip to shoulder and around the star, until all five points of the star have had attention and release. This especially supports our parasympathetic nervous system. (13)

The six-pointed star is actually more accurately described as two interlaced triangles with one pointing upward to the occipital ridge at the base of the head in back, and the forehead in the front. The other triangle points downward to the sacrum and pubis. One very restorative posture is the fetal position presented in chapter 2. Here we curl up on our left side, with the right hand resting on the sacrum and the left on our forehead. With closed eyes, we can relax as long as we need to, letting the nervous system release and restore as we breathe, relaxing from the parasympathetic nervous system all the way to the sympathetic. (14)

Star Patterns Within Us

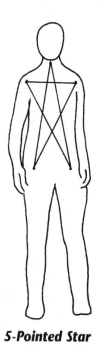

5-Pointed Star

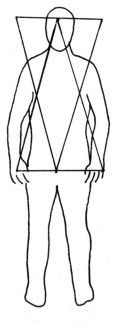

**2 Interlaced Triangles
(Sometimes called
6-Pointed Star)**

ENERGETIC NUTRITION: ACID-ALKALINE BALANCE
KEY: foods in italics=on the Purifying Diet

LIQUIDS:	*Blood purifying herb teas,*	**MOST**
	such as dandelion root, nettle, red clover,	**CLEANSING**
	burdock, turmeric, or triphala	
	Vitality Drink: Liver Flush	
	Polaritea	**MOST**
	Fresh wheat grass juice	**ALKALINE**
	Barley green, other young grass drinks	**FORMING**
	Fresh vegetable juices, fresh fruit juices	
	Pure water	
	Clear vegetable broths	
	Spirulina, chlorella, or wild blue green algae	
	drinks (in moderation.) *	
	Unpasteurized apple cider vinegar *	
RAW	*Fresh fruits and vegetables*	
FOODS:	*Easily digestible raw sprouted seeds, grains,*	
	beans, esp. alfalfa, mung	
	Freshly made vegetable pickles, raw cabbage	**ALKALINE-**
	sauerkraut (homemade, free of sugar &	**FORMING**
	chemicals)	
COOKED	*Steamed leafy vegetables*	
FOODS:	*Steamed root vegetables*	
	Cooked fresh fruits	**MILDLY**
	Cooked sprouted grains, seeds & beans,	**ACID-**
	esp. millet and mung	
	Soaked dried fruits (except prunes &	**FORMING,**
	cranberries)	**BUILDING**
	Grains	
	Legumes, mung is esp. cleansing	
MINIMIZE	*Soaked almonds (up to 8 per day on purifying)*	
IN FASTING,	*Raw honey (small amounts)*	
BETTER	*Essene bread (if fresh)*	
FOR	*Cold-pressed olive or flax oils, other oils*	
BUILDING:	*Avoid corn oil (thyroid inhibitor)*	
	Ghee (heated fat)	
	Potatoes, cranberries, plums, prunes	
NOT	Raw goat milk	
FOR	Other raw nuts & seeds	
FASTING,	Raw cheeses	
	Raw nut & seed butters	**MORE**
DESIGNED FOR	Nutritional yeast, vinegar, pickles	**BUILDING**
BUILDING OR	Fish, poultry, eggs	
GOURMET	Cooked cheese & dairy, breads, tortillas,	
VEGETARIAN	chapattis, roasted nut & seed butters,	**MOST ACID-**
	baked goods with oil or butter cooked	**FORMING**
	into them	

(7) This chart is loosely adapted with permission from Paul Pitchford, *Healing with Whole Foods*, revised edition, p. 240, for use with Polarity diets, with appreciation to him.

*=in excess, the high protein blue-green algae and green algae can be acidifying

ALKALIZING FOOD FOR PURIFYING: (cont.)

Fresh Vegetables

acorn squash	jicama	
artichoke	kale	
arugula	kohlrabi	
asparagus	lettuce	
beans, snap	mache	
bean sprouts	mizuna	
beets	mustard greens	
broccoli	okra	
Brussels sprouts	onions, leeks, chives	
burdock root	pac choi	
butternut squash	parsley	
cabbage, all kinds	parsnips	
carrots	peas	
celery	peppers	
celtuce	purslane	
chicory	radicchio	
collards	rutabaga	
cucumber	shallots	
daikon radish	snow peas	
dandelion greens	spaghetti squash	
& root	spinach	
endive	sprouts of all kinds	
escarole	squash of all kinds	
fennel	tomato	
fenugreek sprouts	turnip and greens	
and greens	zucchini	
garlic		
green beans		
greens of all kinds		
Jerusalem artichoke		

Sprouted Grains Only

millet (especially
alkalizing)
quinoa
amaranth
buckwheat
rice

Sprouted Legumes Only

aduki
mung
other
beans
in moderation

Soaked & Sprouted Nuts and Seeds

almonds
(eight per
day usually)
sesame
sunflower

*Eat as often as you are hungry, and drink as much Polaritea
   as you like
* Breathe deeply.   * Rest.   *Move.
* If you can, get some Polarity bodywork.
* End of the day: Rest, go to bed when you're tired.

VITALITY DRINK: LIVER FLUSH:

Combine well in a blender:

6 oz. fresh orange, apple, or grapefruit juice
1 Tbsp. fresh lemon juice
1 Tbsp. cold-pressed olive or almond oil
1 inch fresh ginger root, peeled and chopped
1–2 cloves garlic (optional)
cayenne to taste (optional, use with caution)

(8) This recipe follows closely one given in *Murrieta Hot Springs Vegetarian Cookbook*. The variations on ingredients and the explanation of dynamics are my own.

Follow immediately with a cup or two of Polaritea:

POLARITEA:

Bring to a boil:
4 cups pure water

Add:
1/2" fresh ginger root, coarsely chopped
1 Tbsp. fennel seeds
1 Tbsp. fenugreek seeds
1 1/2 tsps. licorice root
1 Tbsp. flax seed

Cover and simmer all ingredients over low heat for 10-15 minutes, or turn off heat and steep 30 minutes or more.

Add:
1 Tbsp. dry or small handful fresh peppermint

Steep another 10 minutes or so, strain, and drink.

DYNAMICS, LIVER FLUSH

fresh fruit juice: alkalizing
fresh lemon: strongly alkalizing
olive oil: stimulates discharge of bile from liver
almond oil: more calming if there is inflammation, such as colitis
ginger root: stimulates digestion and circulation
garlic: rich in sulfur, detoxifying to liver
cayenne: cuts mucus

DYNAMICS, POLARITEA

ginger: warming, anti-oxidant, stimulates digestive fire
fennel: neutral energetic, clears gas, supports digestion & weight loss
fenugreek seeds: warming, strengthens digestive fire, builds tissues
licorice root: cooling, anti-inflammatory, soothing, laxative, brings out the best qualities of the rest of the spices, holds fluids in the body
flax seeds: laxative, builds immunity and ojas, helps membranes transmit a healthy charge from one part of the body to another
peppermint: cooling, digestive

These are the distilled modern recipes that are often used for Polarity Purifying. And yet it is interesting to look at Dr. Stone's original prescriptions, which follow:

ORIGINAL VERSIONS OF DR. STONE'S LIVER FLUSH:

TAKE ONE:
1–3 Tbsps. of pure, cold-pressed almond or olive oil
3–9 Tbsps. of fresh lime or lemon juice.

Stir together, drink. Follow with:

2 cups hot water with juice of 1/2 to 1 lemon in each cup.
(9)

TAKE TWO:
1–3 Tbsps. of pure, cold-pressed almond or olive oil
1 cup FRESH orange, grapefruit, pomegranate, or pineapple juice.
Follow again with the two cups of lemon water
described above.
(10)

TAKE THREE:
3–4 Tbsps. of pure, cold-pressed almond, olive or sesame oil
6-8 Tbsps. of fresh lemon juice (about a cup)
Add:
fresh ginger juice to taste.
"If you can get grapefruit, add the juice of one grapefruit or several oranges, and drink it."
"Chew and swallow three to six small cloves of garlic with the oil mixture. Then have the hot tea mentioned above without sweetening."
(11)

ONE ORIGINAL VERSION OF STONE'S POLARITEA:

Take two or more cupfuls of hot herb tea made of:
Licorice Root
Himalayan Mountain Violet
Anise or Fennel
Peppermint
Fenugreek

At the time of serving add:
fresh lemon juice
fresh ginger juice to taste
honey if desired ("Do not use honey with the liver flush.")

If constipated, use more licorice root and fresh garlic.

If experiencing diarrhea, use no licorice, ginger, or liver flush. Instead, use cinnamon sticks in the herb tea. Blackberry juice is also useful here. (12)

ABOUT THE LIVER FLUSH:

In recent years I find some younger students in need of more care for their livers, especially those dealing with higher levels of toxins concurrent with compromised livers. In this situation, the regular liver flush may stimulate queasiness or nausea. If this is the case, instead of the liver flush, begin by substituting the juice of half a lemon in a cup of pure warm water on rising instead. If even this stirs nausea uncomfortably, try plain hot water on rising for a week or more, up to a month. If this is well-tolerated, the lemon in hot water can be tried again. If this sits well over a one to two week period of daily use, a mild liver flush such as the Vitality Drink recipe given here, can be tried again. Fresh air, exercise, and reducing dramatically the intake of chemicals, intoxicants, recreational drugs, and stressful emotional conditions helps tremendously in these situations.

CLEANSING SUPPORTS:

Checking your own tongue is an easy Ayurvedic way to assess the relative need of your gut for cleansing. If there is a thick coat throughout the tongue, ama (waste) has accumulated throughout the gastro-intestinal tract. If there is a coat toward the back of the tongue, the waste has primarily gathered in the colon, the large intestine. Usually the coat will be white. If it has a yellowish hue, the liver is also in need of support and cleansing. As you follow a cleansing diet, whether Purifying or Health-Building, relative to your needs and past food choices, you can watch the changes on your tongue. Often more waste will accumulate for a few days, as it is being released into the digestive tract. This can be reflected by an even thicker coat on your tongue. Then, as the waste breaks down and is eliminated through your colon, your tongue will start to clear up. You can help this process along by gently scraping the coat off with a spoon or tongue scraper.

Fifty years ago, Dr. Stone recommended a colon cleanse which could be done at home in the bathroom simply by flushing shower water up the rectum. Today, what city water would be pure enough to be able to do such a technique safely? And yet one can do enemas with purified water, bastis (Ayurvedic enemas) with herbal teas or oils, or various laxatives or colon cleanses. Standard dosages are about one tablespoon of herb per cup of boiled water, then strained very well. For example, in Ayurveda, one tablespoon of triphala per cup of pure water is steeped, then put through a cheese cloth folded about eight times or so in a tea strainer. You want to get any powder or leaf residue out of the enema preparation, or it can clog up your application bag at some very inopportune moment. Temperature is also important, comfortable to the skin being best; teas cool down quickly.

In terms of perspiration and the skin, Dr. Stone's salt glow (chapter 1) is an excellent cleanser during a fast. Simply showering is helpful, because as we release toxins through the skin, they need to be washed away. Otherwise, we may simply reabsorb them.

Again, in cleansing the air element, it is important to give ourselves chances for deep breathing in fresh air during our cleanse.

It is important to consider how you will create a respite for your nervous system and mind as well as your body during this fast, as they usually get much stimulation in this world. These systems run on glucose, about 60 grams minimum of this simple carbohydrate each day. To minimize uncomfortable sensations, like headache, weakness, or nausea related to low-blood sugar, you want to give yourself enough glucose for the nervous system and brain to function happily. Some of us have abundant fat supplies that in this sort of situation can be converted into glucose for fuel. Some of us don't. For those in the second category, water fasts can be overly heroic ventures. Sixty grams of carbohydrate is equivalent to 240 calories, or about 2 1/2 apples, 1 1/2 oranges, a cup of carrot juice, or 6 cups of steamed kale. Remember to feed yourself as you fast.

If your adrenal glands are exhausted, in most cases you will need to build before you can consider cleansing.

THE CURRENTS AS CLEANSING SUPPORTS:

Polarity bodywork, Polarity chi gung and Polarity yoga (see chapter 2) all activate the flow of the currents, enabling accumulated congestion to clear out. It is important to combine breath with these for maximum beneficial effects.

Working with the transverse current supports our nervous system and our ability to relax and take in breath. Supporting the spiral current strengthens our digestive fire and helps clear old waste out of the digestive tract. Balancing the long lines is a potent way to free long-held emotional patterns and equilibrate each of the five elements flowing within the long lines.

STARS WITHIN US:

Polarity offers additional support for the nervous system in two geometrical patterns of bodywork release. They are called the five-pointed star pattern and the six-pointed star pattern. The five-pointed star connects our shoulders, hips, and head. If we stand up with our legs shoulder-width apart and stretch our arms straight out at our sides, we can see this star pattern in ourselves, like a giant starfish, as we did in some of the movements in chapter 2. A tremendous amount of nervous tension can be stored in this pattern, in the pelvis, shoulders, and neck. Receiving a Polarity Therapy bodywork session can be quite supportive during a cleanse. We can also work the pattern ourselves, with one hand massaging and holding the neck while the other works around the hip. Then we can work shoulder to hip, opposite hip to shoulder and around the star, until all five points of the star have had attention and release. This especially supports our parasympathetic nervous system. (13)

The six-pointed star is actually more accurately described as two interlaced triangles with one pointing upward to the occipital ridge at the base of the head in back, and the forehead in the front. The other triangle points downward to the sacrum and pubis. One very restorative posture is the fetal position presented in chapter 2. Here we curl up on our left side, with the right hand resting on the sacrum and the left on our forehead. With closed eyes, we can relax as long as we need to, letting the nervous system release and restore as we breathe, relaxing from the parasympathetic nervous system all the way to the sympathetic. (14)

Star Patterns Within Us

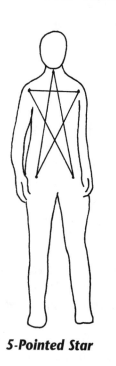

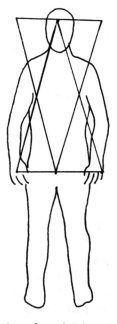

5-Pointed Star

2 Interlaced Triangles (Sometimes called 6-Pointed Star)

ABOUT FAT:

The thing to remember about fat cells these days is that they form a depository. Yes, I know, you groan. Yet fat cells offer more than a refuge for new fresh fat. Fat is a haven for heavy metals and "organic" (that is, carbon-based) chemicals. As we burn up fat, we release stored toxins, far more than most ancestors of a hundred or five hundred years ago.

Appallingly enough, our nation is doing the same thing in its cement manufacturing: when the raw ingredients of cement are incinerated, some companies have managed to get permission to burn up toxic wastes at the same time, including plutonium and dioxin. As concrete is manufactured in these plants, plutonium and dioxins are released into the air around the factory. You can imagine how that would feel to a community located next to such a plant. And similarly, you can imagine how your body could feel, as the fat cells start to release their loads. So even if you think you have an ample supply of fat to get yourself through a cleanse, it is worth taking it easy. Go slow and drink plenty of water, because the generous amounts of fat can also hold generous amounts of toxins. In this situation, you especially need to baby each of the organ systems discussed earlier, the colon, the kidneys, the skin, the lungs, and the brain and nervous system. For more information about environmental toxins, see CLEANSING AND THE ENVIRONMENT.

OPTIMIZING FOR SUCCESS:

To be successful in a personal cleanse, it's worth taking the time to customize your plan to best suit your own needs. In all cases, it is wise to choose as pure and restful a place and time to fast as you can create. You will need psychic space, as well as physical space and time, to be able to do a healing fast. For example, if you are a single mom with a full-time job, don't try it until you have both free time and childcare, even if it is for just one miraculous day or weekend.

The best time to cleanse is usually at the change of seasons, especially spring and fall. Anytime between spring and fall can also be helpful. Generally it is best to avoid fasting if the weather is cold or unsettled, as it can aggravate the doshas more than it helps them. If you are familiar with your constitutional type (see chapter 1), here are some additional tips for making your cleanse as easy and effective as possible.

FASTING AND THE CONSTITUTIONAL TYPES:

AIR TYPES: Short cleanses are best, especially your first one. You would be wise to fast with food. For example, you could choose a Polarity Purifying process that included both raw and cooked foods with the Polaritea and the liver flush. You can balance your selection of airy foods like lemons and oranges with more grounded root vegetables, sweet potatoes, and small amounts of avocado. A first cleanse might last from one to three days. A person experienced in cleansing might use purifying foods for five days or more. It's okay to eat as often as you are hungry. Fresh papaya juice in place of orange juice in the liver flush may sometimes feel more appropriate for you; it stimulates digestion. Munching on papaya seeds is an ancient Ayurvedic way to clear out worms. (15)

Take the time to rest. Let yourself notice when you are tired, and slow down. This process is here to help you heal, not run you down. If you are a thin person and your weight or energy drops dramatically, you can always return to the Health Building process (see chapter 7) to stabilize. If the weather is cold, focus more on freshly cooked foods, less on raw ones. If you skip any meals entirely, skip no more than one or two, maximum.

Flax seeds, up to four tablespoons per cup of hot water steeped, promote colon cleansing. They are also a rich source of essential fatty acids and protein, nourishing to your tissues. Soaked almonds and sprouted sunflower seeds provide relatively benign snacks if you're feeling hungry and in need of grounding. Sprouted mung beans cooked up into soup with vegetables can offer the experience of a "real meal" when you're needing it.

Food combining is important. Fruit needs to be eaten by itself. Take it easy on raw apples, pears, and cranberries. You might want to experiment with baked apples, cooked in fruit juice. Often they are a comfort food, and a rich source of pectin, fiber cleansing to the colon. Soak any dried fruit you use in pure water until it is moist and tender. Hot packs, hot baths, steam, oil massage, Polarity bodywork, and Polarity Yoga and dance would all be great to do if you feel ready for them. Pancha Karma, the Ayurvedic cleanse, is another excellent way for air types to clear out old waste.

FIRE TYPES: Short to medium length fasts work well, as long as your blood sugar stays steady. With stable blood sugar metabolism, a fire type could try one to three days of cleansing with fresh juices (see Dr. Stone's CLEANSING HOME REMEDIES table for specific suggestions.) If your glucose regulation tends toward hypoglycemia, many of the suggestions for the air type also suit you, such as more frequent meals, solid foods, enough protein foods like the sprouted mung, almonds, and sunflower seeds. Like the air type, begin by skipping just one meal, breakfast, having the liver flush followed by Polaritea. You can follow this a few hours later when you get hungry with fresh vegetable juices of your choice.

It's also a fine idea to fast with food, using the Purifying Diet and raw as well as cooked fresh foods. You can make your fast with nearly all raw foods in hot summer weather if it suits you. Emphasize sprouted seeds and legumes (mung beans are especially detoxifying), dark leafy greens (nettles are great in the spring for the kidneys, if you can get them), cilantro, fresh and dried grass drinks like wheat grass, barley green and so forth. Take it easy on oils, hot spices, very sour fruits, and avocados. You may find that fresh apple juice in the liver flush feels better to you than orange.

Checking in with your liver via your mood can be a practical way to monitor yourself: Are you feeling ferocious? Use the smaller amount of olive oil in the liver flush, and cut back or eliminate the garlic in it. You can use ginger for the stimulating spice in the liver flush in place of garlic. It won't have as cleansing an effect on the liver, yet it will stimulate digestion in general without riling your mind as much as the garlic does. Are you getting enough fresh air and exercise? This will also help clear and strengthen your liver, when done in the cool of the day, and help your mood.

If you have a history of stomach ulcers, it's important to take it easy on the garlic and cayenne, or avoid them entirely. Slippery elm tea, extra licorice in your Polaritea (or just plenty of Polaritea in general), mint, fennel, and cilantro are all calming in this situation.

Psyllium seed, one tablespoon per 12 ounces of cool pure water or fresh apple or pear juice, acts as a good laxative. Dry brush massage, cool plunges, fresh air, Polarity Yoga and dance, Polarity bodywork, and deep breathing all help you keep cool.

WATER TYPE: You can do long fasts, if you feel ready. Pure water, rest, and movement are all essential for your success. Following the Purifying food process with an emphasis on watery foods like greens, summer squashes, fresh vegetable juices is excellent. You can begin the day with the liver flush and Polaritea; you may find you prefer a little less licorice root in the Polaritea than most, as one of its attributes is that it is moisturizing and helps hold water in the body. Edgar Cayce's Three Day Raw Apple Fast, especially with organic Golden Delicious apples, rich in cleansing pectin, can work well for your type. You could handle an all-raw diet if you like, or you can add in some fresh cooked foods. You can emphasize diuretic foods, if this feels warranted: sprouted adukis, sprouted millet, sprouted amaranth, fresh parsley, and carrot juice. Easy on items like Essene Bread, honey, fructose (which I don't recommend for any type during a fast), excess oil, and avocados. Flax seeds, one to three tablespoons in ginger tea, acts as a good laxative. Chia seeds are good for energy. The time limit to your fast is dependent on you, your body, and energy. I have seen some water types cleanse on a purifying process for 3 weeks or more, and simply feel better. If this is your first time for a cleanse, even a day can feel good.

Emotions are likely to come up (see processes in chapter 8). Give yourself time for creative expression, such as writing, journaling, painting, or dancing. Let your feelings flow, no need to hang on to them. You may appreciate a good friend reflecting back to you what you're saying and feeling, to get some clarity on the "below-the-belt" issues that could emerge. On the other hand, you may just feel good and happy; that's normal, too.

Let yourself spend time in or near pure running water, if you can. And drink as much pure water as you want to consume. If you have the budget, seaweed wraps can be excellent for you, at the local spa. Like the Earth Type below, bitter, pungent, and astringent tastes in foods will support the deepest cleansing of your tissues.

EARTH TYPE: All that has been written above about the Water Type applies to you, too. You can undertake as long a fast as you (and your trusted health consultants) feel you capable of doing. Raw foods and fresh juices are excellent for you, including fresh apple juice diluted one to one with pure water. You might want to peruse Dr. Stone's CLEANSING HOME REMEDIES chart for further ideas about the best fresh vegetable juices for you. The one exception to this focus on raw foods and beverages would be if the weather were icy. Then it's smart to go more for fresh cooked foods. Plenty of light is important to nourish your tissues. Regular or spontaneous exercise, deep breathing, pranayama, Polarity bodywork, Polarity Yoga, saunas, and steams, any or all of these are beneficial for you during this time. Balance your use of root vegetables with light, leafy greens as well. Working in the earth with your hands can be revivifying. You might even want to play with mud or clay packs, or bury yourself in sand! These processes with the Earth help draw out toxins for you.

In terms of tastes, as much healthy bitter (greens, fresh herbs), pungent (ginger, garlic, fresh herbs, chiles), and astringent (asparagus, sprouted legumes) tasting foods as you're willing to consume will stimulate deeper cleansing.

APPLYING THE GUNAS IN POLARITY PURIFYING:

When you're purifying, if the food is fresh, organic, and lovingly prepared, you will cleanse more thoroughly, as well as more easily. This means the sattvic category of foods will serve you well during a cleanse. Most tamasic foods are especially important to avoid when clearing out parasites. Yet Dr. Stone used some specifically rajasic and tamasic herbs or plants in his cleanses, for particular advantages. The liver flush has a powerfully active effect on this organ. Garlic, rich in sulfur, pulls out heavy metals, essential in detoxification. It is rejuvenative, and stimulates the digestive fire of each of the seven tissues (dhatus). It is also hot, pungent, aggressive, and heating to the mind. It can aggravate an ulcer. If you find yourself becoming more ferocious on the liver flush than is comfortable for <u>you</u> to handle, you can consider dropping the garlic and using ginger alone in the flush for its digestive stimulating effects.

Likewise, Dr. Stone used onions on the Purifying program. Roasted onion can be especially useful in grounding your energy if you're feeling spacey or disoriented. It can cut down your meditative focus and increase desire, so there are trade offs here, depending on your priorities. It can be a helpful anchor.

DISCOVERING A BALANCE IN PURIFYING

Obsessions can go too far. At the peak of my passion for cleansing, I was inspired to help our chickens eat more "purely". After all, I was cleaning up my act, why not they? When they finished off their last bag of commercial lay pellets with the reputed dead animal flesh inside, I began feeding them a mix of organic grains. I was respecting the purity of the Sacred within them, but—without reference to what they needed physically. After a month on this "pure" diet, they looked ratty, were increasingly irritable and fussy, and their egg laying was waning. Instead of bringing out their innate beauty and strength in some deeper way, I had unwittingly run them down physically. (I was not so naive as to imagine they were experiencing a "cleansing crisis"; we'd had chickens a while.) Now their "pure" diet includes more of everything they need, including extra protein (soy meal and fresh milk) and vital minerals (kelp powder) along with the grains.

I've had friends whose way to be vegetarian was McDonald's drive-up, hold the burger. Cheese and bun, right?

I began to think, are chickens so different from us? Of course, yes, they are. And yet, often we get some mental idea of how we're supposed to be eating, without referring or deferring to commonsense physical need. (I guess we have more ideas than chickens do.)

Some of us need more protein than others, doubly so if we're growing ourselves, growing a child, nursing a child, or recovering from an illness, especially an illness that involves long-standing inflammation or fever. At times like these, a purifying diet is not appropriate.

CLEANSING AND THE ENVIRONMENT:

Usually when we choose to cleanse, we have some good cause for deciding to do so. Perhaps we sense generally that our immunity is compromised, or we are working with a specific life-threatening illness such as cancer. The mass media in this country strongly encourages us to look at the development of illnesses in terms of our own life-style choices and genetics, when it covers issues like reduced immunity or cancer. And yet, for example, recent medical statistics suggest that 80% of new breast cancer diagnoses are women with no family history of the same. Smoking is a crucial carcinogen, aggressively marketed all around us. Yet most carcinogens are released in a blanket of silence. The total global production of synthetic chemicals, a good percentage of them petroleum-based, has increased from one billion pounds in 1940 to over 600 billion pounds in 1990. That's 300 million tons of chemicals. To pretend that this is not a major factor in health or cleansing would be more than naïve.

While I have talked about fresh air, pure water, good food, and clean soil, much of what we have access to these days is not. Being a self-care text, the focus has been lifestyle choices we make. And yet to make clear choices, we need solid information. The mass media, in collusion with other industries and government in the U.S., provides little of this when it comes to topics like chemicals, cancer, and immunity. Physician Samuel Epstein has crusaded for decades for full disclosure from industry and government as to what chemicals released into the environment do, in us as individuals and in us as communities. In a recent interview, he was asked what we can do about this proliferation of chemicals. His responses were action-provoking. The first action he recommended was "the vigorous pursuit of the 'right to know'." The second was to "ban new hazardous technologies." Third, he advised phasing out "a variety of hazardous products and processes already on the market."

Dr. Epstein points to some small spots of hope in the large dirty picture. For example, in 1989 consumers and industry worked together to get the state of Massachusetts to pass a Toxic Use Reduction Act, which has successfully phased out the use of most of the nastier organic solvents, replacing them with safer alternatives. Some large businesses, such as Xerox, the copy machine king, and Interface, a major carpet supplier, are creating more ethical business practices, choosing to responsibly lease and recycle their products, rather than randomly leave them to be dumped in the environment, as many companies do. Major pharmaceutical companies and computer producers are obvious places on which to focus a long-overdue recycling spotlight.

Rather than be depressed at the magnitude of the problem, Epstein encourages us to wake up and focus on prevention and clean-up. The impetus will have to come from us rather than multi-nationals concerned more about profits than health, he says; it is to our immediate advantage to discover more about what is going on in our communities and workplaces. A succinct and clear-minded individual, Dr. Epstein has written a number of books of interest, including *The Breast Cancer Prevention Program* (Macmillan, 1998), *The Safe Shopper's Bible* (1995), and the prize-wining classic, *The Politics of Cancer* (Sierra Club Books, 1978). He was an advisor to the European Union in their successful choice not to allow in the import of hormone-contaminated meats. (16)

What would you focus on, if you were to come up with one environmental toxin to clear out of your home or community?

ABOUT USING THE HOME REMEDY TABLES:

Dr. Stone described numerous home remedies that one could use on one's own, or in conjunction with the three food processes. Some of his vast body of recommendations is presented here for your information in the following CLEANSING HOME REMEDIES tables. These tables are distilled directly from his teachings and writings, undiluted with other perspectives, other than an occasional editor's note. They run the gamut from lemon and oil rubs to self-perineal work. Many fine techniques have been omitted, simply because they need more space to communicate or they seem difficult to convey on paper to someone new to the techniques.

From this compilation I hope to stimulate us to a wider use of appropriate therapies and further research into Stone's methods. It would also be useful to know when NOT to use these remedies. There is an opportunity here to research these recommendations further. Some of the recommendations are extensive; others are brief. I don't believe any of them has been assessed clinically in any systematic way: that is their risk as well as their opportunity. If you have any questions about any procedure, check-in with a trusted health care practitioner before trying it. An open mind and some good common sense will come in handy as you explore these. There is the potential for major rebalancing in these processes. On the other hand, there is also the chance that a process or remedy could create problems for you, if followed for too long or with too much zeal. This information is a quirky and inspiring look at healing. It offers no substitute for your own knowledge about yourself and what you need.

I present this information with some trepidation, in that much of it is taken out of context, and it is but a small fraction of what Polarity self-care is. Often a demonstration is an easier way to communicate a process than written words. While I am reporting Dr. Stone's work directly in these tables; it is important to realize that much of what is reported here I have had little or no experience of using. Dr. Stone's approach to nutrition is very different from my own. I believe that here the spotlight needs to be on his work, so that we can clearly see what the origins of Polarity Therapy are, as it develops in this new century and millennium.

LOOKING AT ONE CONDITION: OSTEOARTHRITIS:

I would like to explore one condition a little more thoroughly here to give encouragement in using these succinct charts more extensively on your own. Looking for "osteoarthritis" under *BONES AND JOINTS* in the Home Remedies chart, you will find a few specific recommendations from Dr. Stone. These include drinking fresh carrot, celery and cabbage juice as a purifying practice, running cold water over the affected joints while rubbing them to stimulate circulation, a daily morning liver flush, a strict vegetarian diet without starch, and as much purifying food as you can muster. Each of us is different, with different needs and metabolic rates, and so none of us will respond to these recommendations in exactly the same way. However the mere simplicity of them warrants further explanation. Much of what Dr. Stone offered was deceptively simple, and often extremely useful.

So, look at these recommendations step-by-step. Carrot juice is extraordinarily rich in potassium, from 500 to 1,500 mgs. per cup, while celery is a good source of natural sodium, 150 mg per cup of the raw vegetable. Figures are not available for celery juice, yet one could estimate that a cup probably offers 600 mg of sodium or more. Cabbage juice is a fine, if not very tasty, source of vitamin C, without the irritating effects on the joints that many vitamin-C- rich foods like citrus can have. Frequently in osteoarthritis there is an underlying condition of adrenal fatigue. These three juices support the adrenals effectively, giving them the potassium, sodium, and vitamin C they may be needing. When the adrenals are in good shape, they make natural anti-inflammatories for us, our bodies' equivalents of cortisone. When the adrenals are tired, they often fall behind in their job of providing the body with an adequate supply of anti-inflammatory hormones, or begin to make an unbalanced supply. This deficit can aggravate the joints.

These juices also are alkalizing to the kidneys, promoting cleansing. The kidneys (along with the liver) are the major organ sites where toxic metals are stored in our bodies. Vitamin C helps begin to clear these out. An accumulation of heavy metals can be behind certain kinds of osteoarthritis and joint stiffness. For example, an excess of aluminum has been correlated in one British study (17) with hip pain and stiffness. Lead can also have an adverse effect on the joints; this is a common component of the air breathed in many large cities.

The cold-water rinses are especially useful when the right wrist pulse is weak and the left pulse is relatively strong (see chapter 8 for further information about the pulses).

The Polarity Liver Flush helps relieve toxic accumulations in that organ; again, these can be heavy metals, pesticides, insecticides, dry-cleaning chemicals, and other industrial exposures. It also stimulates cleansing of the bowels, of particular help in relieving pain in the lower back.

The strictly vegetarian, non-starch diet has interesting effects. This is generally a purifying diet, without any bread, grains, pastries, tortillas, potatoes, eggs, cooked oils, or heated dairy. In essence, it cuts out most of what might clog us up, intestinally. Yet it also eliminates the meat and potatoes, both literally and metaphorically. It acts essentially as an allergy-elimination diet, if done for five days or more. If you want to use it this way, eliminate all grain for at least five days. Then you can add one grain back in one day at a time after your purifying time is over. For example, you might add in wheat on the first day after the purifying process, amaranth or quinoa the next, rice the next, corn the next. You may find that some of them contribute to your stiffness. More and more, an allergic component is being recognized in the treatment of arthritis. Eggs are another potential offender here. If you have followed Dr. Stone's program faithfully for a length of time, eggs are not part of your diet. But for many readers, eggs may be a common food that either agrees with them famously or, surprisingly, contributes to joint pain. Four days on the purifying diet without eggs is usually enough to reveal if they are a problem for you.

Usually digestive stagnation contributes to allergies, and the Purifying program with the liver flush begins to rebalance that. There is another factor here, with starch and arthritis. Even if you are not allergic to any grain, blessedly, you may be harboring an excess of the bacteria *Klebsiella*. This microorganism has been garnering more attention in recent years, because a build-up of it in the large intestine has been, unusually enough, correlated with joint pain. The recommended remedy? A low-starch diet, because *Klebsiella*, like *Candida*, has been found to proliferate with an excess of starches. (18)

Your build and your personal health history will dictate whether these recommendations are useful short-term or long-term. For those of us with a history of excess, including excess weight, the Purifying process may feel good for a longer length of time, since it helps relieve pain as well as shed weight. For the scrawnier, malnourished, adrenal-fatigued types among us, a strict vegetarian diet may only contribute to bone-deep fatigue and pain if followed for too long. In recent years, adequate protein intake has been associated with better bone health and osteoporosis prevention.

CHAPTER SYNOPSIS:

CLEANSING:

What kind of house cleaning do you need to do?

Physical?

Emotional?

Mental?

Spiritual?

Are you willing to create the time and space
and conditions to do the kind of cleansing you need?

RESOURCES IN CLEANSING:
BOOKS:

Stone, Randolph, *Health Building.*

Buist, Robert, *Food Chemical Sensitivity: What it is and how to cope with it*, from an early pioneer on the subject.

Chakravarti, Sree, *A Healer's Journey*, uses touch, yoga, mantra, and color in healing, written by a East Indian woman elder.

Gagnon, Daniel and Amadea Morningstar, *Breathe Free: Nutritional and Herbal Care For Your Respiratory System*, hones in on common respiratory ailments, with a physiological explanation of each illness.

Galland, Leo, *The Four Pillars of Healing*, written by a Western physician especially skilled at working with difficult digestive problems.

Joshi, Sunil V., *Ayurveda and Panchakarma: The Science of Healing and Rejuvenation*, excellent in-depth discussion of both the theory and practice of this ancient science.

Lad, Vasant, and David Frawley, *The Yoga of Herbs: An Ayurvedic Guide to Herbal Medicine*, excellent specifics on cleansing herbs.

Leichnitz, Will, RPP, The Polarity Training Institute, 566 Pharr Rd., Atlanta, GA, 30305, strong understanding about working with the three nervous systems in healing.

Murrieta Foundation, *Murrieta Hot Springs Vegetarian Cookbook*, an abundance of delicious American-style vegetarian recipes.

Perera, Sylvia Brinton, *Queen Maeve and Her Lovers: A Celtic Archetype of Ecstasy, Addiction, and Healing*, a powerful look at addictions and change from a wise Jungian.

Pitchford, Paul, *Healing with Whole Foods*, classic text integrating Western and traditional Chinese nutrition, from a therapist deeply skilled in cleansing techniques.

Tiwari, Maya, *Ayurveda: Secrets of Healing*, includes many traditional Pancha Karma techniques from an author who has used Ayurveda in a deeply healing way in her own life.

ABOUT CANCER: Here are several books I find myself recommending often:

Kushi, Michio, with Alex Jack, *The Cancer Prevention Diet.*

Lerner, Michael, *Choices in Healing: Integrating the Best of Conventional and Complementary Approaches to Cancer.*

Weed, Susun, *Breast Cancer, Breast Health.*

EDUCATIONAL PROGRAMS:

Frawley, David, *Ayurvedic Healing Correspondence Course for Health Care Professionals*, Santa Fe, 1996, American Institute of Vedic Studies, PO Box 8357, Santa Fe, NM, 87504-8357, phone: (505) 983-9385, fax: (505) 982-5807, www.vedanet.com, email: vedicinst.@aol.com. This course provides a thorough grounding in the basics of Ayurvedic healing, including in-depth information on the dhatus.

POLARITY CLEANSING RETREATS IN NATURE:

(partial listing, please check with APTA for updated listings, (303) 545-2080, email: SATVAHQ@aol.com).

Bruce Burger, MA, RPP, offers the Polarity Cleansing Diet as a nine day personal retreat annually in mid-July, on 240 acres of wilderness in northern California, with pool, sauna, hot tub, and nourishing community life. Contact Heartwood Institute Ltd., 220 Harmony Lane, Garberville, CA 95542, phone toll-free: (877) 408 WOOD (9663) or (707) 923-5005, 923-5000, http://www.heartwoodinstitute.com.

Polarity Wellness Center of Vermont offers two Polarity Cleansing Retreats each year, spring and fall, in a rustic, beautiful wooded area with creek, adjoining national forest land. Contact Suellen Trumbour Cheney, RN, RPP, office: 228 Main Street, Ludlow, VT 05149, (802) 228-2136. The Polarity Wellness Center of Vermont also offers other opportunities to learn about Polarity Therapy in nature, in co-operation with Carol Ann Lucia and the Energy Healing and Polarity Center of Woodbury, Connecticut.

SUPPLIES:

Heretical suggestion: for those of us who wish we could just take an alkalizing pill, here's a possibility: Ormed, Inc. is a nutritional company supplying health professionals. It offers an effective alkalizing capsule for short-term use, Alkabase. They are working on a citrate-based product for longer use. PO Box 1021, Forestville, CA 95436, phone (707) 575-7070, fax (707) 887-1715.

CLEANSING HOME REMEDIES FROM DR. STONE: 1

BODY SYSTEM & Condition	HOME REMEDY:	OTHER RECOMMENDATIONS FROM STONE ON THIS CONDITION:
BLOOD PRESSURE **Hypertension (high blood pressure)**	Fresh celery, beet and carrot juice, daily (1)	1) Garlic can be added to the fresh juice, if you are brave. 2) Purifying diet. 3) Hot baths with cold rinse, followed by an oil rub. (2) 4) Stretches which stimulate the spinal muscles, drawing energy out of the congested core to the periphery. (3)
Hypotension (low blood pressure)	Fresh carrot, beet and dandelion juice While sitting, gently knead your abdomen in a clockwise direction to release stagnation and gas.	1) Here, avoid full hot baths & hot water to the spine. Instead, use warm baths with several cold rinses. (4) 2) Apply hot packs to the abdomen. 3) Polarity touch: Place your right hand on your feet, your left on your belly as long as you like. Then, bring the energy up from your feet toward your head with "relaxed hands". (5)
BLOOD SUGAR **Diabetes**	Fresh carrot, celery, string bean, and Brussels sprout juice, 8 oz. 3x per day	More fresh raw food. Avoid all white sugar and artificial sweeteners. Millet is preferable, as it is alkalizing and protein rich.
BLOOD VESSELS **Phlebitis**	Fresh celery, beet and carrot juice*	
Varicose veins	Fresh carrot, spinach and turnip juice	

CLEANSING HOME REMEDIES FROM DR. STONE: 2

BODY SYSTEM & Condition	HOME REMEDY:	OTHER RECOMMENDATIONS FROM STONE ON THIS CONDITION:
BONES AND JOINTS **Arthritis, osteo**	Fresh carrot, celery and cabbage juice	1) Use the morning liver flush daily and "adhere to a strictly vegetarian, non-starch diet". 2) Purifying diet with alfalfa sprouts. (7) 3) Run high-powered cold water over the affected joints for twenty minutes twice per day, gently rubbing them as you do. 4) Check pulses; often they are strong on the left indicating over-extension, see chap. 8. (8)
Arthritis, rheumatoid	Juice of half a lemon before each meal and before retiring, to alkalize the system. Otherwise, avoid citrus. (OK to use other fruits in the liver flush.)	1) Morning liver flush. (9) 2) "Strictly vegetarian, non-starch": purifying diet. 3) Reduce gas, avoid fermentation at all costs. Ex: avoid acid-starch combinations like OJ & toast, as well as heated oils. (10) 4) Make generous use of alfalfa &/or fenugreek sprouts, and dark leafy greens. (11) 5) Take it easy on sour drinks like kefir & buttermilk, store-bought yogurt, and rich foods. (12) 6) As in osteoarthritis, run cold water vigorously with a hose on the affected joints for twenty minutes twice per day, gently rubbing the joints as you do. See also pulse, above.

CLEANSING HOME REMEDIES FROM DR. STONE: 3

BODY SYSTEM & Condition	HOME REMEDY:	OTHER RECOMMENDATIONS FROM STONE ON THIS CONDITION:
BONES AND JOINTS (cont.) Back pain	Work sore spots on tops of feet (if you can reach them). Put one hand on the sore spot in your back, the other on the top of the feet Hold until you feel a therapeutic pulse. (gentle throbbing in rhythm in both areas) or otherwise feel more relaxed, less pain. Do as often as needed.	1) Hot sitz baths as needed for pain relief. 2) Strict vegetarian diet, with more green leafies and fruits, less animal protein. (13) 3) Hot & cold showers, alternating, ending with cold. 4) Mustard plaster or cayenne ointment rub to the affected areas. 5) See also (14) perineal tx. 6) Work the "psoas magnus-iliacus plus" points on the outside of each foot, and/or the "psoas magnus" points on the base of each thumb. See Chart # 17 which follows this table.
BREASTS Swollen	Lemon juice compresses, with equal parts fresh lemon & cold water, as needed. (15)	
Congestion, lumpy breasts		For discussion of the relationship of congestion in the breasts with the calves, backs of knees, buttocks, & upper back, see (16).
CANCER, in general	Avoid frequent use of over-heated fats.	Stone saw cancer as a pre-eminently cold, watery disease, and recommended avoiding water foods like celery and cucumber. (17)

CLEANSING HOME REMEDIES FROM DR. STONE: 4

BODY SYSTEM & Condition	HOME REMEDY:	OTHER RECOMMENDATIONS FROM STONE ON THIS CONDITION:
G.I. TRACT **Cirrhosis of the liver**	Peel a lemon, chop it, cover it with honey and eat it.	1) Start with one lemon a day and increase to as much as ten lemons per day (rinse mouth well after each, ed.). Increase one lemon each day until improved, then "work backwards down to one a day." (18) 2) Avoid alcohol. (19) 3) Follow a fruit and fresh juice diet while on this regime.
Colitis	Almond oil is recommended when doing a liver flush for this condition. (20)	See Chart # 17 following: work the "eliminative" and "ascending colon" points on each hand, regularly.
Constipation	Fresh cabbage, spinach, celery, and lemon juice. Squats are an excellent stretch. For specifics, see (21).	1) Plenty of fluids, & adequate oil: even as much as 1/2 cup olive, almond or sesame oil with 1/2 cup fresh lemon juice, four times per day (!) (22) 2) Purifying diet, including generous amounts of fenugreek & alfalfa sprouts. 3) Liver flush. (23) 4) Add pears to your green salads. (24)
Diarrhea	Fresh grated apple mixed with lemon juice, cinnamon & a little honey. (25)	1) Do not do liver flushes. 2) Use no licorice or ginger in the Polaritea, instead substitute cinnamon sticks. 3) Use blackberry juice. 4) Drink cinnamon steeped in rice and/or barley water. (26)

CLEANSING HOME REMEDIES FROM DR. STONE: 5

BODY SYSTEM & Condition	HOME REMEDY:	OTHER RECOMMENDATIONS FROM STONE ON THIS CONDITION:
G.I. TRACT Flatulence (gas)	Chew well. Food combining is important; simplify your food choices at each meal. If you're eating beans, try sprouting them for greater ease of digestion. Squatting, a few minutes each day, strengthens digestive function substantially. (27)	1) For more specifics of food combining, see *Health Building* (28). Avoid drinking liquid with your meals, unless it is a little fresh ginger juice, or ginger-fenugreek-peppermint tea. Sprout beans before you cook them to enhance digestibility. Prepare cabbage family vegetables with ginger and black pepper. 2) Avoid over eating. 3) Shoulder stretches: the more flexible your shoulders are, the less gas accumulates. (29) 4) Work on the fleshy part of each thumb. See Chart #17 which follows.
Gallstones, &/or sluggish gallbladder	Fresh carrot, beet & cucumber juice.*	Also, chew the seeds of lemons, grapefruit and oranges well, 5 minutes or more. (30)
Gastritis	Fresh carrot, celery & cabbage juice.	See Chart #17, digestive-pylorus-stomach line.
Hemorrhoids	Fresh carrot & parsley juice.*	1) Liver flush. (31) 2) Silver ring on left little finger.
Liver, sluggish	Liver flush. Specific bodywork, see (32).	Easy on sugar and starch. Avoid heated oils.

CLEANSING HOME REMEDIES FROM DR. STONE: 6

BODY SYSTEM & Condition	HOME REMEDY:	OTHER RECOMMENDATIONS FROM STONE ON THIS CONDITION:
G.I. TRACT *(cont.)* **Spastic bowel, dry**	1 Tbsp. olive oil with 1 Tbsp fresh lemon or lime juice several times per day.	Follow with plain hot water and "use a fruit diet for a few days." (33) Work on the fleshy part of the thumb and the outside of the feet; see Chart # 17.
HEAD **Headaches**	Purifying diet with water and fresh papaya until the pain passes. The focus here is to reduce any excess gas build-up. There is an extremely useful Polarity technique for relieving headache, see (34).	1) Avoid liquid with meals, especially cold drinks. 2) Notice the food combinations you've made prior to the onset of the headache. You can try avoiding these combos in the future, to see if this helps. 3) Avoid fried foods. 4) Work your toes gently, then firmly. Esp. focus on any sore spots.
REPRO-DUCTIVE SYSTEM Impotence	Keep gonads cool: alternate cold & hot running water on them.	*"Discard the jockstraps and tone the tissues."* (35)
Menstrual cramps	Perineal work can be very helpful.	For more information, see (36).
Prostatitis	Hold inside heel of both feet.	Specific squat, see (37).
Vaginal discharge	Douche with fresh lemon juice in boiled pure water.	"In varying amounts" , as needed to relax and soothe tissues. (38)
RESPIRATORY SYSTEM Adenoids, swollen or infected	Fresh carrot, beet* & tomato juice.	*"Lemon & oil sniffed up through the nose...clears up adenoids."* (39) Work along the upper ridge of the fleshy part of the thumb, see chart #17.

CLEANSING HOME REMEDIES FROM DR. STONE: 7

BODY SYSTEM & Condition	HOME REMEDY:	OTHER RECOMMENDATIONS FROM STONE ON THIS CONDITION:
RESPIRATORY SYSTEM (cont.) Asthma	To calm tense lungs, try this Polarity hold: right hand on abdomen, left on forehead, while sitting. Also, cold wash cloth on upper back for 5 minutes at a time.(40) Repeat these several times.	1) Follow a starch-free, milk-free diet. See also all recommendations for bronchitis. 2) Use fresh lemon or lime juice, 2 Tbsps. before each meal & at bedtime. (41) 3) Squats, with side-to-side or circular motion. (Ed. note: see also good stretch, the Rocking Cliff, in chap. 2, done 5 minutes daily.) (42)
Bronchitis *"and all catarrhal (mucus-filled) conditions"*	Fresh carrot and radish juice.	Avoid cream, ice cream, starches, sugars, and eggs. Simplify food combinations, especially avoiding protein-starch combinations. (43) To open up the sinuses & airways, try this: mix 4 oz. of grated horseradish with 2 oz. of lemon juice, 1 tsp. garlic juice, & 1 Tbsp. honey. Take a tsp. or more of this mixture four times per day. (Ed.: my guess is this is to be taken orally, not nasally.) See Chart # 17 for reflexes.
Colds and coughs	Fresh lemon or lime juice with pineapple juice, honey, & water, before & between meals, & at bedtime.	1)"Some garlic" can be added to the juice combo. 2) Avoid cold, wet feet: it aggravates lymphatic flow to the head. (44) See Chart #17 following.

CEANSING HOME REMEDIES FROM DR. STONE: 8

BODY SYSTEM & Condition	HOME REMEDY:	OTHER RECOMMENDATIONS FROM STONE ON THIS CONDITION:
Sinusitis	Scissor kick, see Polarity Yoga routine, chap. 2.	Squatting, working the inside of the mouth with your thumb. (45)
RESPIRATORY SYSTEM (cont.) **Sore throat**	Use lemon juice & almond, olive or sesame oil as a gargle. Take it internally as well.	If there is swelling, try lemon juice compresses to the area, with equal amounts of lemon & water. See also "colds". (46)
Tonsils, inflamed or infected	Fresh carrot, beet* & tomato juice.	
SKIN **Abscesses and eruptions**	Take lemon with oil internally, almond, olive or sesame.	Topically, use a poultice of lemon pulp on the skin. (47) (Ed. Note: if line appears running from abscess, get medical attention immediately.)
Athlete's foot	Apply fresh lemon juice & fresh papaya juice to the skin. (48)	
Boils and carbuncles	Apply hot flaxseed poultices to the area. (49)	1) Fresh carrot, beet* & celery juice. 2) Fruit diet to assist elimination. 3) Easy on rich foods. See also "abscesses".
Eczema	Apply almond or olive oil with fresh lemon juice to the area. And drink the same. You can also try fresh lemon juice with pineapple juice applied externally until the skin is clear.	Follow a starch-free, all-fruit diet which includes lemon and oil. (50)

CLEANSING HOME REMEDIES FROM DR. STONE: 9

BODY SYSTEM & Condition	HOME REMEDY:	OTHER RECOMMENDATIONS FROM STONE ON THIS CONDITION:
SKIN General health of skin	Baking soda and salt rub to skin in the bath. Use twice as much baking soda as salt on a wet soapy washcloth.	Follow with a warm rinse, then a cool rinse, then a light oil rub all over. Towel dry. (51)
Pimples	Fresh carrot, beet* and celery juice.	
Scalp, general tonifying, and for infections	Massage fresh lemon juice & olive or almond oil directly into the scalp. (52)	
Temporary food stains, odors, or discolorations on the hands	Rub the hands with the pulp and rind of a lemon that has already been juiced. (58)	
Wrinkles, especially under the eyes	Gently massage a mixture of fresh lemon juice & olive or almond oil from the out-side of the eyes inward toward the nose. "Also, from the same outer corner of the eye in an upward diagonal direction."	(54)
TEETH & GUMS Pyorrhea, or to clean discolored teeth	Rub a combination of lemon juice and salt into the gums, several times a day (55).	(Ed. note: rinsing well recommended.)

CLEANSING HOME REMEDIES FROM DR. STONE: 10

BODY SYSTEM & Condition	HOME REMEDY:	OTHER RECOMMENDATIONS FROM STONE ON THIS CONDITION:
URINARY TRACT **Kidney stones**	Fresh carrot, beet* & cucumber juice.	Easy on alcohol. Gently work the "kidney reflex" area on the outside of each foot. See Chart # 17 which follows.
TOXICITY *(in general)*	Purifying diet.	Craniosacral work. (56)
OTHER ISSUES: Condition		
ADDICTIONS & HABITS **Alcoholism**	Have the following Vitality Drink when craving alcohol: Blend 1 cup of alfalfa or fenugreek sprouts with pineapple juice and honey. Take as needed.	1) Health Building diet. 2) Avoid meat, fish, eggs, & heavily spiced foods. 3) Suck on a lemon when you have craving for alcohol. (57)
Tobacco	Suck on a lemon when craving arises, as often as you need to, for a month or more.	Same as above: eliminate meat, fish, eggs, heavily spiced foods.
FATIGUE **Low energy with thirst**	Vitality Drink (see above).	
Sluggish mind, under-stimulated	Breath through your nose, not your mouth.	Wear a gold ring on your thumb and a silver one on your big toe. (58)
Sluggishness, physical	Eat supper light and early; avoid late heavy meals.	Stretch: the Wood Chopper. (59) (Ed. note: CAUTION: LOWER BACK)

CLEANSING HOME REMEDIES FROM DR. STONE: 11

OTHER ISSUES Condition	HOME REMEDY:	OTHER RECOMMENDATIONS FROM STONE ON THIS CONDITION:
Fever	"Give the body a rest from food". Drink hot water with lemon, lime or grapefruit juice, until you feel better. Or sip fresh lemon juice with clover or alfalfa tea. (60)	1) "Milk is a food"; don't eat it now. 2) Keep skin cool & moist with cooling compresses. 3) If fever is very high, 104 degrees or above, cooling enemas can be given to bring the temperature below 104.
Insomnia	Try an evening meal of fresh fruit, with or without warm milk.	Avoid heavy, late meals. Do a few minutes of squatting before bedtime, with your arms around your legs and your head bent down. (61)
Overweight	Purifying diet.	Eat a light supper, "not too late". (62)
PAIN Caused by indigestion, can show up in the calves of the legs, arms, chest, or back		Avoid cooked oils. Follow Health Building diet. (63) Be sure the pain is not from another cause, such as obstructed blood vessels.
Sudden onset of pain, anywhere in the body	"Give the body a rest": see "fever".	

* "The juices of beets, parsley and watercress are very concentrated and should not be used too freely. About four ounces per day, mixed with other juices, is plenty." Stone, *Health Building*, p. 74

CHART NO. 17.   THUMBS AS NEUTER REFLEXES EMBRACING THE ENTIRE AREAS BELOW THE DIAPHRAGM ON EACH SIDE OF THE BODY, COMPARED TO REFLEXES AROUND THE OUTSIDE OF THE ANKLES AS THE NEGATIVE POLE.

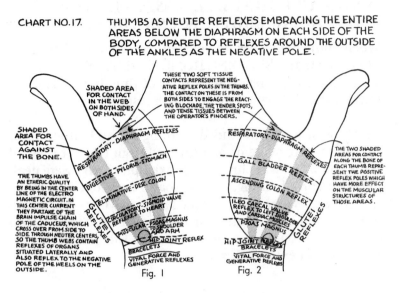

Chart #17: Thumbs. Reprinted from Dr. Randolph Stone, *Polarity Therapy*, vol. I, bk. 2, p. 24, with gracious permission by CRCS Publications.

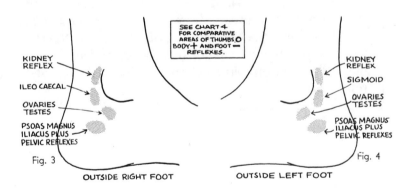

Chart #17: Ankles. Reprinted from Dr. Randolph Stone, *Polarity Therapy*, vol. I, bk. 2, p. 24, with gracious permission by CRCS Publications.

(64)

POST-SCRIPT TO THE CLEANSING TABLES: ABOUT DOING BODYWORK ON YOURSELF:

When doing bodywork on yourself, as recommended in the CLEANSING and BUILDING HOME REMEDY tables from Dr. Stone, there are a few simple rules of thumb. One is don't hurt yourself! Work a sore area with respect.

Dr. Stone also recommended working top to bottom if the condition were acute or painful, and from the feet upward if the condition was chronic. For example, if you were dealing with chronic indigestion and also had cold feet, Stone might begin by shining a heat lamp on your feet. If you were dealing with acute diarrhea and fever, Stone would advise you NOT to use such heat. See the box below for Stone's comments on this.

WORKING WITH ACUTE OR CHRONIC CONDITIONS:

"ALL ACUTE AND PAINFUL CONDITIONS are treated with the current flow, usually from above downward. ALL CHRONIC AND SUBNORMAL CONDITIONS are treated beginning at the extremities (ed.: hands or feet), in an upward and inward direction, to augment the weakened return currents." (65)

VII.

———•———

BUILDING

Rejuvenation and Regeneration:
How to nourish the tissues well.

"Those who are destined to look for true health will find it." STONE, *HEALTH BUILDING, P. 9*

Simple Things We Could Do:

Chew.

Eat when hungry.

Move when restless.

Rest when tired.

The focus in this chapter is on rejuvenation and regeneration. How can we nourish our tissues well? As a nutritionist, I have increasingly come to respect our individual differences when it comes to building a body. Some people do very well with a vegetarian diet, while others seem to do better with some amount of animal meat. I'd like to address both possibilities in this chapter, so that you can rebuild in a way that suits you.

The key to building tissue lies in our digestive fire. Because we must first digest food before we can absorb it into our tissues, healthy digestive fire stands metaphorically as the entryway to rejuvenation. In Ayurveda, a common sense kind of analogy is made. If you imagine a fire, a good solid roaring fire, you can throw all sizes of wood into it, and it will be readily consumed. Yet imagine you have a small fire, just beginning to burn. If you immediately throw a big log on this fire, it will put it out, with lots of noxious smoke, to boot.

When we are babies, we have little fires, and we are fed accordingly: small meals, when we are hungry (hopefully), with easy to digest food. Now we are big people. We assume we have a big fire and can eat everything we want at any potluck in town. Although some of us may have learned at an early age that this is not true, yes? Some of us have a generous amount of this big fire, this digestive fire called agni in Sanskrit, and some of us do not.

Dr. Stone makes a nearly identical analogy for Polarity's approach to digestive fire, in the following quote. *"Food must be digested just as fuel must be burnt, or clinkers remain. If the good reader ever fired a furnace or a boiler in a power plant, he learned a few very valuable lessons, namely:*

1st—Not too much shoveled in at once.
2nd—Spread the coal thinly over the hot embers.
3rd—Regulate the draft.
4th—Select the fuel which will burn best—leaving the least amount of clinkers—with the least fumes and smoke." (1)

In terms of fuel, some of us will make "clinkers", indigestible particles, at the thought of meat and potatoes, while others of us know our bodies balk at beans or dairy, no matter how they are prepared. It is important to have a realistic knowledge of our current choices and capacities.

DIGESTIVE FIRE:

So how can you ascertain the size of your own digestive fire? Your appetite will let you know how strong your digestive fire is, and your tongue can tell you a good deal about your digestive efficiency. When your appetite is strong, your digestive fire is usually strong, too. When your appetite is

strong and your tongue is clear, you are ready to start building, or rebuilding. A clear tongue indicates you are burning
fuel efficiently. A coated tongue suggests you are accumulating ama, incompletely digested waste, otherwise known
as the "clinkers" Dr. Stone referred to above. A primary
indicator of inefficient digestion is also gas. If you are a
hungry person with a good appetite, and you have a thick
coating on your tongue (and perhaps some gas as well),
your GI system needs re-balancing to experience greater
efficiency. Often simpler food combinations are important
here (see FOOD COMBINATIONS chart which follows in this
chapter). You may also want to review the last chapter on
cleansing, given your tongue coat.

You've got a nice clear tongue but little appetite? In this
situation, you need to pay attention to nurturing your digestive fire. This is the first step here. The table below shows
common conditions and how we can respond to them.

DIGESTIVE FIRE AND EFFICIENCY

APPETITE	TONGUE	CONDITION
Strong	Clear	In general, healthy, ready to build or maintain.
Strong	Coated	While your digestive fire is probably strong, your digestive efficiency is foundering some. You may be overeating or eating food-combinations you're not digesting well. The GI tract needs some balancing and cleansing.
Weak	Clear	Need to build digestive fire.
Weak	Coated	Need to eat more lightly, build digestive fire, and clean out GI tract.
Variable	Either coated or clear	There is a need to develop a regular digestive fire. See hints below in ENCOURAGING DIGESTION, especially about regular meals.

As a reminder to readers, in both Ayurveda and Polarity Therapy, if there is a need for cleansing, it is usually done before we build. Otherwise wastes and toxins can move deeper into our bodies, creating potential health difficulties later on.

ENCOURAGING DIGESTION:

From the point of view of Western physiology, adequate digestive fire means secreting appropriate amounts of hydrochloric acid in our stomachs. This acid begins the breakdown of protein foods, essential in building. It also protects us by killing most microbes, viruses, bacteria, and yeast, with its strong acid. In Ayurveda, too, digestive fire (agni) is valued both for its transformative and protective effects. The gut, in Ayurveda, is considered the beginning of immunity, the first line of defense. Many simple practices encourage digestive fire. Here are some essential basics:

Eat your biggest meal of the day in the middle of the day, when digestive fire is likely to be highest.

Breathe in a relaxed way throughout the day. Breath feeds digestive fire.

Eating at regular times of the day encourages a steady digestive fire.

Regular exercise promotes an increase in agni, as long as it is not done right after eating.

Relax and let yourself enjoy the meal.

Eating in stillness encourages digestive fire, as long as you find it relaxing.

Simple food combinations can encourage weak digestion to improve.

The judicious use of spices with meals can help stimulate digestive fire.

Fresh ginger tea is a very good way to encourage digestive fire, sipped with meals. Fresh ginger juice is an even stronger stimulant to digestion.

In Ayurveda, a combination of equal parts of cumin, coriander and fennel seed is drunk as a tea with meals to harmonize digestion.

A smoothly functioning spiral current enhances digestion significantly. (For more about the spiral current, see chapter 2).

Breathing deeply feeds our digestive fire.

WAYS WE DAMPEN OUR DIGESTIVE FIRE, OFTEN UNKNOWINGLY:

Cold drinks douse digestive fire.

Exercising right after eating discourages digestive fire, by drawing blood flow away from the internal organs to our limbs.

Eating on the run is discouraging to long-term agni (digestive fire).

Eating at erratic times is confusing to digestive fire, and can impair its efficiency.

The more sluggish we are, the droopier our digestive fire tends to be.

Eating when we're upset is often challenging to digestive fire.

Eating late at night can heighten digestive inefficiency, because usually digestive fire is lower at this time.

From a Western nutrition perspective, a deficiency of either zinc or B vitamins can lower both appetite and digestive fire.

WEIGHT GAIN AND WEIGHT LOSS IN AYURVEDA:

The ancient Ayurvedic texts view weight gain and weight loss a little differently than we often do today. In Charaka, the frustrating cycle of weight gain is described in the following way. Once we have gained a considerable amount of weight, fat obstructs the channels, trapping vata and then pitta in the abdomen. Appetite increases, and so does digestive fire. As soon as we eat something, it is quickly consumed, and we want more. Unless we can shift this pattern, we grow fatter.

The recommendations of the ancients are interesting as well. A warming diet which calms Vata and Kapha and simultaneously reduces fat is advised, one which is "heavy and non-nourishing" to satisfy the digestive fire without increasing mass. What kind of foods might these be? Those with a lot of fiber, yet few calories, such as plenty of fresh vegetables or oat bran muffins. The Polarity Health Building diet could fit the bill here. In this situation, the channels definitely need to be cleared, and the Ayurvedic cleansing process of Pancha Karma can be quite useful. (2)

In underweight conditions, the view is that slim people need a "light and nourishing" diet. Often here the digestive fire is impaired, either in the gut or the tissues, and trying to eat heavy, complicated meals will be counter-productive. Small frequent meals, soups, stews, adequate protein are some examples of these. At the same time, digestive fire needs to be supported, and the whole being needs to relax. Sharma's translation of Charaka puts it delightfully: "Freedom from anxiety about any work, intake of nourishing diet and adequate sleep make the man fatty like a boar." (3)

Pure water is vital, from an Ayurvedic perspective, in nourishing every tissue, all the dhatus. (4) Often we are dehydrated and do not realize this. If there is headache, back pain, or emaciation, it is worth looking at the amount and purity of the water we are receiving.

Some people find that they feel below par if they fall below a certain weight. In these situations, it is worth contemplating the following quote mentioned earlier from Charaka: "Diseases get automatically alleviated when dhatus are brought to their normal state." (5) In other words, feed yourself adequately, let the nourishment penetrate deep within you, and you will get better.

FOOD-COMBINING FOR ANY WEIGHT REGIME:

When digestion is stressed, simplifying the food combinations you eat can help. The following chart in the Western naturopathic tradition indicates which foods can be digested easily together for most people, and which foods present challenges to a more delicate gut, or one with lower digestive fire. These combinations are based on concepts from Western physiology. In the relative ease of digestion of foods, for example, beans and nuts are both relatively heavy and so are better eaten in small quantities together, or not at all. Other foods, like fruit, digest so rapidly on their own, that they can ferment if contained in the stomach with other foods, causing gas. Still other foods do well on their own, yet inhibit the digestion of another category of foods. A common example here is acid and starch, as in salsa and chips, orange juice and toast, or tomato sauce and pasta. Starch enzymes in the mouth are inhibited in an acid environment, so eating an acid with a starch can slow down the breakdown of the starch. Remembering the concept of okasatmya, if these agree with you, relax. However, if they don't, you may want to simplify.

Food Combining, Polarity

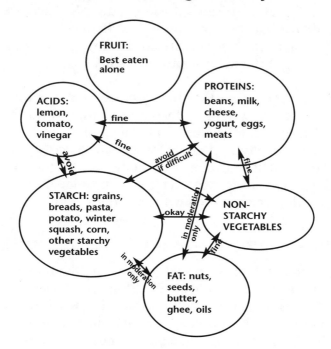

FRUIT: Best eaten alone

PROTEINS: beans, milk, cheese, yogurt, eggs, meats

ACIDS: lemon, tomato, vinegar

fine

fine

avoid

avoid if difficult

fine

STARCH: grains, breads, pasta, potato, winter squash, corn, other starchy vegetables

NON-STARCHY VEGETABLES

okay

in moderation only

fine

in moderation only

FAT: nuts, seeds, butter, ghee, oils

THE POLARITY HEALTH BUILDING PROCESS:

The Polarity health building process builds strong tissue, while giving you a minimum of "grungy" food. It is ideal if you want to build health, and shed some weight in the process. If you are already lean and are following a Polarity program, you may want to combine the health building diet with the gourmet veggie one, to be sure you get enough calories. An Ayurvedic building approach follows this section.

A TYPICAL HEALTH BUILDING DAY:

Wake up, stretch, breathe, enjoy.

Have some fresh water with lemon in it, or some hot Polaritea, or hot ginger tea.

When you are hungry, have something to eat:

Fresh fruit:	Or, warm cooked grain:	Or, a protein:
Any kind you like, especially if it's in season,	Millet, cinnamon oatmeal, brown rice cream, spelt, kamut, hot corn atole, kashi, teff, to name a few	A Spirulina smoothie, steamed tofu "scrambles", a glass of fresh hot (or cool) milk, a bowl of cottage cheese or fresh yogurt, or some fresh soft cheese

AT LUNCHTIME, CHOOSE FROM:

Fresh vegetables:	With a protein:	Or, with a starch:
Any kind you like, especially if it's in season,	Well-prepared beans, like Middle Eastern dal, or hummus, or pinto beans, or adukis or...	Sushi rice, or pasta, pasta with basil, any grain you like, brown rice, wild rice...or...
Fresh sprouts, any kind you like, including alfalfa, sunflower, bean sprouts (mung), fenugreek	Soft cheese or yogurt or milk	Potatoes, baked or otherwise, just not fried or heated in oil
Sea vegetables, like sushi nori, or dulse, or kombu (kelp) or hijiki or arame.	Raw uncooked nuts and seeds, or their butters: tahini or almond or cashew.	Bread or crackers, as long as they have no cooked oil in them: like French Meadow Rye, or rice cakes, or...

Any of this could be served with some tasty dressing, like lemon and olive oil, or basil almond pesto sauce or flax and garlic, just so long as the fat has not been heated up. Ghee is not included in a Health Building regime, as it is a heated oil.

Let yourself digest completely, get back to work or school or play.

When you're hungry, you can choose a snack or two. (If you're not hungry, and your blood sugar is just fine, skip the snack and build digestive fire).

HEALTH-BUILDING SNACKS:

Fresh fruit or veggie:	High-fat protein	Or, a low-fat protein
Any kind you like,	(alone or with veggie:)	(alone or with fruit or
including fresh carrot	Raw nuts or seeds, like	veggie):
sticks, an apple, an	pumpkin seeds or sun-	Fresh dairy, yogurt,
orange, a peach or..	flower seeds or almonds	milk, soft cheese,
	or....	organic preferred
Fresh veggie or fruit		
juice, like carrot or	An almond drink	A soy shake, or baked
orange		tofu

If none of this appeals, think of the carbohydrates: grape leaves with rice (dolmas), corn on the cob, sushi with veggies..... (H'm, we may be into dinner here...)

Dinner uses the same food combinations as lunch, just lighter. For example: brown rice with veggies, hearty soup, baked potato and salad.

GOING GOURMET VEGETARIAN:

You apply the same principles as in the Health Building regime, you just loosen up around the heated oil, nuts, seeds, and dairy. (6) You can use these foods heated as often as your liver can handle them happily. Signs of a potentially unhappy, sluggish liver include the following: one is reluctant to get out of bed in the morning, and yet it is easy to stay up late. Then it is hard to get out of bed again in the morning. One might feel sluggish, depressed, irritable, or headache-y.

THE GUNAS IN HEALTH BUILDING:

Each of the three gunas can be used in your design of a health-building program. Foods from the sattvic category are especially useful if you are rebuilding both your physical and mental health. They are gentle, supportive and clear. Some examples include fresh vegetable soups, fresh milk or yogurt, fresh flat breads and whole grains, fruits, or freshly made smoothies.

Not all of us have the luxury of a sedentary life however, and more rajasic foods serve well when we're doing more strenuous physical work: protein-rich foods like hummus, fresh soft cheeses, or a yogurt from the store. Rajasic health building also includes foods like tofu, soy milk, tempeh, pickles, garlic.

Tamasic food is primarily intended for grounding, when it is used in a conscious way. Onions have been mentioned as stabilizing during a cleanse. Often though, we use tamasic foods unconsciously, to numb out. Who among us hasn't zoned out with a bag of chips or some other such satisfyingly unregenerate trash after a long and intense day? (Yes, that's Veggie Gourmet, not Health Building, right?)

While tamasic foods like these or leftovers or frozen food are not warmly regarded in most Ayurvedic circles, Dr. Stone, at least in some parts of his life, had no problems with them as a category. One friend in Polarity was listening to Dr. Stone on audiotape (rare opportunity!) and reported that the lively gentleman in his single later years advocated a simple dinner of canned peas as the answer to culinary dilemmas!

WHAT ABOUT BEING A VEGETARIAN OR NOT?

In East Indian Ayurveda, being a vegetarian is considered the most ethical way to eat, if you can be healthy doing so. When vegetarian diet is not recommended, it is usually due to health concerns. In Polarity, being a vegetarian is highly valued, yet not all Polarity practitioners these days are. Dr. Stone strongly believed that a vegetarian diet was most optimal both for the efficacy of his Polarity Therapy and his personal spiritual path. At one point in his life, he felt so strongly about this that he reportedly would only work on people who were eating a vegetarian diet. Later, he dropped this requirement. (7)

My concern, as a Polarity practitioner and nutritionist, runs two ways. I see some people running themselves down physically with an unrealistically strict vegetarian diet, while I see others afraid to give up their traditional American diet, rich in animal protein for even a short time for fear of weakness. There is a lot of emotion in both camps. Deborah Madison's latest book, *Vegetarian Cooking for Everyone* offers one potential middle ground. She creates delicious food that treads lightly on our planet's ecological balance, and invites us to eat it as often as we like. Her approach is that anyone can try tasty vegetarian food, and that many of us could benefit from less animal protein. This moderate perspective will not satisfy those of us with deeper urges to purify, and yet in the long run it may get more of us eating in a lighter, healthier way.

Dr. Stone's three food processes can be tremendously healing when utilized in an appropriate way, for an appropriate length of time for the given individual. They can in fact be profoundly supportive of spiritual meditative processes, as many practitioners have found. And yet I find students of Polarity today often let themselves get psyched out by the supposed intenseness of the process, and so choose to miss out on a process that is best learned through doing. It is definitely possible to do these processes in healthy, safe ways and get the results you are after.

For some long-term practitioners struggling with poor health after thirty years of vegetarian diet, it is worth investigating why Ayurveda does not always recommend a vegetarian diet for everyone at all times. The key lies in the relationship between the doshas, the gunas and ojas. A sattvic vegetarian diet is most calming to the mind for most people. And yet for some, especially those who have air (Vata) strong in their make-up, more grounding foods may be necessary to maintain a healthy physical balance. For some, this could be as simple as roasted onions. (And I appreciate that some readers may have taken monastic vows that eliminate this option, too.) For others, it could be a bowl of homemade chicken soup. For others of us, it may be an occasional hamburger, hopefully eaten with deep appreciation for the four-legged whose life was given for that burger.

Why do I single out Vata dosha, air, here? It is cool, light, and dry. When it builds up in excess in the body, it can begin to dry out the moist energy cushion, which surrounds and protects us. This cushion, *ojas*, is vital to our immunity and peace of mind. If it becomes thin, our health can suffer and our sensitivity to input—sounds, bright lights, touch, aromas, taste—can become agonizingly intense. While vegetarian diet is considered best for building ojas for most people, it does not always calm Vata enough to protect ojas from its drying effects. Subsequently, animal foods are sometimes recommended in Ayurveda as medicines. (8) Devotion, rest and time by or in running water helps as well.

Yet, in regard to meat, as Ayurvedic physician Robert Svoboda put it dryly once, "The law of karma has not been retired." (9) In Ayurveda, meat is recommended to save a life and restore health, with a full awareness that you are incurring a debt to that animal you are eating. (10)

The Gunas, Doshas, and Ojas

If Vata increases excessively, ojas is depleted.

Sattvic food builds ojas and prana, as long as Vata is in balance and the food is well-digested.

Rajasic food builds energy and enthusiasm, yet can increase Pitta.

Tamasic food has different effects, depending on the individual's makeup. Some tamasic foods, like onions or meat, ground Vata well. This has the ultimate effect of protecting ojas in the high-Vata person.

Excessive tamasic food increases Kapha and ama. Processed or frozen tamasic foods do not usually help Vata, instead they can create a sense of fatigue, heaviness, or lethargy.

AYURVEDA AND BUILDING:

In Ayurveda, *rasayana*, or rebuilding the tissues, can have a wider intention than just this moment and this life. The intention of rasayana is to strengthen your whole line, your offspring, their offspring, down through the generations, so that your descendents can enjoy better health. (11) There is an awareness in Ayurveda that what we do has a consequence to others in the future. On a purely nutritional level, this view is supported by Western nutrition. Some studies indicate that the nutritional deficiencies of one generation may take as many as three generations to rebalance. In other words, if your grandfather was badly magnesium deficient, you may have a tendency toward that as well, unless your parents fed both you and themselves quite differently.

On a global level, the consequences of ignoring the generations to come have become blatant and painful. For example, pollution has become so widespread that some predict, based on current trends, that European males will be completely sterile by the year 2010, and that American males are only a few years behind them! Whether such dire predictions are exactly on target, it highlights the fact that a radical clean-up is due. (12) Other species have already paid for the consequences of our acts.

If you wish to begin to personally cleanse and build, there are a number of good books about Ayurvedic nourishment (see the RESOURCES section following chapter 5 on Nourishment, especially). What I would like to share here is that you can use specific foods to nourish specific tissues, and it is usually best done under the guidance of an astute Ayurvedic physician. She or he can monitor your tissues for you, so that you do not build up an excess in one area and a deficiency in another.

AYURVEDIC BUILDING PRACTICES FOR THE DHATUS

DHATU	SUPPORTING DOSHA	BUILDING PRACTICES
plasma (*rasa*)	Kapha	pranayama
blood cells (*rakta*)	Pitta	pranayama
muscle (*mamsa*)	Kapha	oil massage
fat (*meda*)	Kapha	rest, contentment
bone (*asthi*)	Vata	specific medicated ghees*
nerve & marrow (*majja*)	Kapha	rest, peaceful atmosphere, specific medicated ghees *, aromatherapy
reproductive: female (*artava*)	Kapha	oil massage, specific medicated ghees*, respect, devotional practices
male (*shukra*)	Kapha	same as above: oil massages, specific medicated ghees, respect, devotional practices

* See Appendix, Personal Self-Care Recipes

ABOUT BUILDING THE DHATUS:

In Ayurveda, food builds each dhatu. When a particular essential dhatu has been properly nourished, not only does it pass nourishment to the next dhatu, it also feeds secondary tissues, called *upadhatus* (see next page). For example, skin is an upadhatu of muscle. This means that if you want to create vibrant skin in Ayurveda, you need to have healthy muscle. So exercise, which is cleansing to muscle, would be part of a healthy skin program, along with adequate protein and other foods to nourish mamsa and oil massages (the right kind for your skin! See *Ayurvedic Beauty Care* by Melanie Sachs, for specific information about this.) Another example: if you are having troubles with your teeth, use bone-supporting regimes. And so on.

AYURVEDA: BUILDING THE TISSUES

Building foods & practices

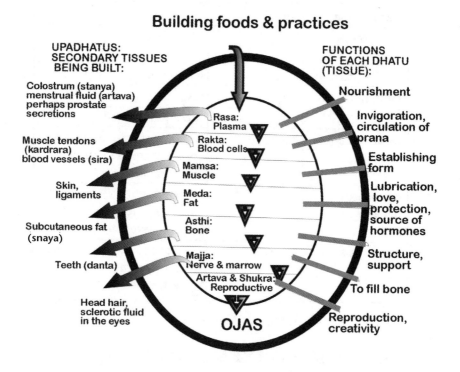

UPADHATUS:
SECONDARY TISSUES
BEING BUILT:

Colostrum (stanya)
menstrual fluid (artava)
perhaps prostate
secretions

Muscle tendons
(kardrara)
blood vessels (sira)

Skin,
ligaments

Subcutaneous fat
(snaya)

Teeth (danta)

Head hair,
sclerotic fluid
in the eyes

FUNCTIONS
OF EACH DHATU
(TISSUE):

Nourishment

Invigoration,
circulation of
prana

Establishing
form

Lubrication,
love,
protection,
source of
hormones

Structure,
support

To fill bone

Reproduction,
creativity

Rasa:
Plasma
Rakta:
Blood cells
Mamsa:
Muscle
Meda:
Fat
Asthi:
Bone
Majja:
Nerve & marrow
Artava & Shukra:
Reproductive

OJAS

BUILDING occurs as each tissue increases in health and vitality.
Five days are needed to nourish each tissue, from the plasma inward.
After absorption from the digestive tract, nourishment goes first to the
plasma for 5 days, then to the blood cells (days 6-10), and so on. It
takes an average of 30-35 days of healthy eating to nourish the
reproductive level. If there is a healthy excess of nourishment at the
reproductive level (rather than simply ama, waste) the body converts
this excess nourishment to ojas, our energy cushion and immunity.

AYURVEDA: BUILDING FOODS FOR THE DHATUS WITH VEGETARIAN DIET

DHATU	BUILDING FOODS FOR EACH DHATU
plasma (*rasa*)	Pure, easy to digest, sattvic foods: enough pure water, almond rejuvenative milk (ARM), fresh raw organic cow's milk, saffron rice and other rice dishes, ghee, kichadi, sweet & sour fruits & their fresh juices, sesame seeds, Recharge-style drinks
blood cells (*rakta*)	Pure slightly sour and salty foods, & those rich in iron & B vitamins: figs, raisins, black grapes, black cherries, blackberries, dates, beets, beans, esp. tur dal & red lentils, pistachios, umeboshi plum, miso, molasses, ARM, saffron milk, sesame seeds
muscle (*mamsa*)	Easy to digest proteins and grains, esp. wheat if it is well-tolerated, also spelt, kamut, millet, corn, other grains, dals, fresh milk, lassi, ARM, urud dal with chapatti, banana followed with ARM 1-2 hours later, ghee, avocado, sesame
fat (*meda*)	Foods rich in essential fatty acids (EFAs), pure heavy rich foods, sweet foods, includes flax, borage, evening primrose oils, almonds & other nuts, ARM, fresh milk, ghee, banana, sesame, coconut, avocado, yam, potato
bone (*asthi*)	Foods rich in minerals that are also easy for Vata to digest: sesame seeds, feta & other pure cheeses, pure dairy of all kinds, wakame, kombu (kelp) & other sea vegetables, ARM, quinoa, teff, amaranth, urud & tur dal, okra, well-cooked dark leafy greens with olive oil or ghee, if well-tolerated, winter squashes, sweet potato (this last eaten alone)
nerve & marrow (*majja*)	Moist whole foods rich in EFAs, vitamin E, & B complex: sesame seeds, almonds, ARM, other nuts, esp. pecan, pinon, walnut; banana, ghee, oats, fresh milk, if well-tolerated
reproductive: female (*artava*)	ARM, sesame seeds, fresh milk, ghee, figs, dates, saffron, cherries, pomegranate (in moderation), banana, oats, tofu, walnuts, Jerusalem artichoke, chickpeas, okra
male (*shukra*)	Fresh milk (highly recommended), ARM, banana, honey, licorice, onion, chickpeas, walnuts, oats, okra, almonds, sesame seeds, ghee, cream

Note: For other building herbal options, see HERBS TO BUILD THE DHATUS chart which follows

AYURVEDA: BUILDING FOODS FOR THE DHATUS
WITH OMNIVOROUS DIET

DHATU	BUILDING FOODS FOR EACH DHATU
plasma (*rasa*)	All of the above in the VEGETARIAN DIET, plus chicken soup, turkey, meat broths, fish soups
blood cells (*rakta*)	All of the above, plus: organic meats (esp. beef), poultry, fish
muscle (*mamsa*)	All of the above, plus: meats, esp. organic beef
fat (*meda*)	All of the above, plus: pork esp., duck, other fatty animals, organic
bone (*asthi*)	All of the above, plus: venison, organic bone in slow-cooking soups
nerve & marrow (*majja*)	All of the above listed in VEGETARIAN DIET
reproductive: female (*artava*)	All of the above, plus royal jelly, bee pollen, eggs, mutton, venison, clean shellfish (avoid bottom-feeding species)
male (*shukra*)	All of the above, plus royal jelly, bee pollen, some eggs, mutton, venison, clean shellfish (avoid bottom-feeding species)

Note: There are many other building herbal options, see HERBS TO NOURISH AND BUILD THE DHATUS chart which follows

In the ancient texts, these recommendations were made with few qualifications, other than it was important to respect the animal and that one ate animals primarily as medicine, to save or restore a life. Other qualifications or understandings are added now: for example, while pork will definitely fatten you up, it is said to clog the channels, srotas, badly. Or, while adding a bone in soup is considered a definite builder for bone in the body, it is also said to toxify the blood. Other food prescriptions relate to differences in opinion among Ayurvedic physicians about specific foods and building tissue. For example, pumpkin seeds are highly regarded as an anti-parasitic food in Ayurveda. In the West, due to their rich zinc content, they are often recommended to strengthen the prostate. Yet some Ayurvedic physicians believe pumpkin seeds weaken *shukra*, male reproductive tissue.

HERBS TO NOURISH AND BUILD THE DHATUS
(Caution: these could increase ama if present)

DHATU	Potent sattvic herbs	Potent sattvic herbs	Potent sattvic herbs	Milder sattvic herbs
RASA (PLASMA)	Amalaki Angelica Bala Bhringaraj Fenugreek Flax seed	Hawthorn berry Licorice Lotus seed Shatavari Slippery elm Rehmannia	Sandalwood Fo-ti Gokshura Tulsi basil Saffron Vamsha rochana Wild yam	Alfalfa Chamomile Chrysanthemum Coriander Marshmallow Raspberry leaf Rose
RAKTA (BLOOD CELLS)	*Saffron* Amalaki Angelica Bala Bhringaraj Fenugreek Flax seed	Hawthorn berry Fo-ti Gokshura Gotu kola Licorice Lotus seed Manjishtha	Rehmannia Shatavari Solomon's seal Sandalwood Tulsi basil Vamsha rochana	Alfalfa Chamomile Chrysanthemum Coriander Marshmallow Rapberry leaf Rose
MAMSA (MUSCLE) includes organs	Ashwagandha Bala Amalaki Fenugreek (liver, lungs, urinary tract) Elecampane (lungs)	Fo-ti Hawthorn berry (heart) Licorice Rehmannia (kidneys & liver)	Sandalwood Saffron Shatavari Vidari-kanda Wild yam Angelica	Chamomile Coriander Marshmallow Raspberry leaf
MEDA (FAT)	Amalaki Aswagandha Bala Fo-ti	Licorice Saffron Sandalwood *Aromatherapy*	Shatavari Vidari-kanda Wild yam	

KEY: *in italics* = especially effective

HERBS TO NOURISH AND BUILD THE DHATUS (cont.):

DHATU	Potent sattvic herbs	Potent sattvic herbs	Potent sattvic herbs	Milder sattvic herbs
ASTHI (BONE)	Amalaki Angelica Ashwagandha Bala Bhringaraj	Flax seed Fo-ti Gokshura Licorice Manjishtha	Saffron Sandalwood Shatavari Solomon's seal	
MAJJA (NERVE & MARROW)	Bala Sandalwood Ashwagandha Angelica Bhringaraj Amalaki Fo-ti Gokshura	Gotu kola Jatamamsi Elecampane Fenugreek Lotus seed	Rehmannia Saffron Shatavari Tulsi basil Vamsha rochana Vidari-kanda Wild yam Licorice	Chamomile Chrysanthemum Marshmallow Rose
ARTAVA (FEMALE REPRO-DUCTIVE)	Shatavari Aswagandha Amalaki Angelica Bala Elecampane Fenugreek Fo-ti	Jasmine Licorice Musta Lotus seed Sandalwood Solomon's seal	Flax seed Tulsi basil Rehmannia Saffron Vidari-kanda Wild yam Gokshura	Marshmallow Raspberry leaf Rose
SHUKRA (MALE REPRODUC-TIVE)	Ashwagandha Shatavari Amalaki Bala Flax seed Fenugreek Gotu kola	Licorice Lotus seed Fo-ti Gokshura Saffron Rehmannia Kapikacchu	Vidari-kanda Wild yam Tulsi basil Sandalwood Vetiver Solomon's seal	Marshmallow

Note: most of this information is derived from *The Yoga of Herbs,* by Drs. Lad and Frawley, with much appreciation for the guidance of David Frawley. Any errors are my own.

Most of the building herbs available tend to be sattvic. Yet there is one herb which is quite rejuvenative to all tissues, and yet is rajasic. This is garlic. So while garlic is excellent for rebuilding, one needs to be aware that it can irritate the mind.

Ultimately, each person must decide for themselves what goes onto their plates and into their mouths. As Dr. Stone said (13) *"It is the <u>essence</u> in the food which we really crave. The gross particles must all be expelled or they would accumulate and we could not carry on. The gross forms are but conveyors of the life essence within them." "Intelligence and the experience gained by the trial and error method act as a safeguard for each person. Rules do not apply equally to all ages nor times, to the same person, nor to every temperament and individual. Mere chemistry does not take into account each person's ability to digest and assimilate foods. That is an individual problem which can easily be proved by every one who is interested enough in his or her well-being to observe <u>what agrees best at what time of day and in what quantities.</u> It is simple but it needs close attention and some unbiased observation which every person should give himself in order to remain well under the stress of work."*

These charts about building the tissues can be used as a guide for those wanting to explore building further from this perspective, either as vegetarians or omnivores. In Ayurveda, one can also build from the outside in. Ghee is infused with rejuvenative building herbs in concoctions known as *ghrtas*. These ghrtas can be taken internally, yet they can also be rubbed on the skin. In the recipes section in the PERSONAL SELF-CARE RECIPES appendix, you can find one bone-building ghrta (without the bone).

ABOUT ESSENTIAL FATTY ACIDS AND BUILDING CHARGE IN POLARITY:

In a Polarity Therapy session, the transmission of charge along a membrane is an essential part of the healing. Nutritionist Udo Erasmus has made the following important observation about essential fatty acids (EFAs), "EFAs help maintain the fluidity of membranes. They also help create electrical potentials across membranes which, when stimulated, generate bioelectric currents that travel along cell membranes to other cells, transmitting messages." (14) When we are well-nourished, charge builds and moves easily. When we are deficient in essential fatty acids or their supporting nutrients (protein, magnesium, zinc, B complex) it is more difficult for a charge or message impulse to be sent from one part of the body to another. Flax, hemp, evening primrose, borage, and black currant oils are all rich sources of essential fatty acids. They can be taken internally, uncooked, or applied topically on the skin. Adequate protein intake seems to be also important for normal EFA metabolism, according to Barry Sears, author of *The Zone Diet*, and can reduce our need for expensive supplemental oils. (15)

WHAT ABOUT BLOOD TYPES?

As a nutritionist, I am often asked this question. I think there could be something to it, and it is not the whole picture. Naturopath Peter D'Adamo has looked at interactions within the blood to define nutritional needs in his best-selling book, *Eat Right for Your Type*. There are well-documented medical differences between the four blood types. How accurate Dr. D'Adamo's specific food recommendations are, remains to be seen over time.

The blood type O's among us do seem to need more protein, usually animal, though not always. There may be subsets among the blood types, as Ayurvedic physician Robert Svoboda has suggested, which have adapted to other conditions. (16) In interviewing a number of long-time vegetarians, including those who had been exclusively vegetarian for twenty years or more, I found a significant number of healthy individuals who were type O. The key to good health in these vegetarian type O's seemed to rest on the following: 1) they made sure to get enough protein, including milk and eggs in their diets, 2) they made a point to do regular seasonal cleanses, at least twice a year, and 3) they lived with an appreciation for Mother Nature and her cycles. Adding more ancient grains to the diet, such as quinoa, teff, or amaranth, and less wheat and corn may also help type O's.

Most blood type A's (not to be confused with heart-risk type A personality, an entirely different term) do seem to do well on vegetarian regimes, as Dr. D'Adamo hypothesized. However, I've spoken with a few type A's who believed that periodic consumption of meat was helpful for boosting their energy levels. Since type A has a documented tendency toward pernicious anemia, caused by deficiencies of vitamin B-12 or folic acid, they may have a point, since meat is rich in these. (Dark leafy greens, cow's milk, cheese, and eggs are other good sources.) I suspect type A's choosing not to be vegetarian would find seasonal cleansing important. If they adjust the lightness of their meals to their digestive capacity on a regular basis, they are also likely to benefit. Realistically, most of us would benefit from one to two seasonal cleanses per year, healthy or not.

It's important to key in on individual needs, and not assume that all of the recommendations given in the Blood Type diet are accurate for you personally. I have seen type B's who needed more animal protein, and other B's who seemed to need less. I've also seen type B individuals with milk allergies, despite the hypothesis that type B handles dairy most easily. I haven't seen a large enough sample of AB's to be able to observe anything useful here. And yet, as a nutritionist, I have had to notice the generous number of people who have mentioned to me positive experiences with this particular approach.

In general, it is one measure that takes into account one factor. It does not take into account our age, environment, changing conditions, digestive fire, or ethical questions. (17) (18) Still, it can be helpful, if we can adapt it to our specific needs and personal choices.

Whatever you are eating, do you want to eat with a full appreciation of the gift of what it is you are consuming?

CHAPTER SYNOPSIS:

BUILDING:
Where are your challenges:

digestion

plasma

blood cells

muscles and organs

fat

bones and joints

bone marrow and nerves

reproductive system

immunity, ojas?

What simple measures could you take to build support for these areas?

RESOURCES IN BUILDING
Books:

D'Adamo, Peter, *Eat Right for Your Type*, for direct information about this system of eating according to blood type.

Johari, Harish, *The Healing Cuisine: India's Art of Ayurvedic Cooking*, many tasty recipes keyed for the doshas.

Lad, Usha and Vasant, *Ayurvedic Cooking for Self-Healing*, with delicious vegetarian recipes according to the doshas.

Lad, Vasant, and David Frawley, *The Yoga of Herbs: An Ayurvedic Guide to Herbal Medicine*, Lotus Press, Twin Lakes, WI, 1986, much specific information on herbs to cleanse and build.

Morningstar, Amadea, *Ayurvedic Cooking for Westerners*, keyed for eating with the doshas.

Morningstar, Amadea and Urmila Desai, *The Ayurvedic Cookbook*, keyed for eating with the doshas.

Murrieta Foundation, *Murrieta Hot Springs Vegetarian Cookbook*, The Book Publishing Company, Summertown, TN, 1987, many good Polarity recipes.

Spignesi, Angelyn, *Starving Women: A Psychology of Anorexia Nervosa*, a Jungian approach which might open your mind to other ways of looking at this process.

Svoboda, Robert, *Prakriti: Your Ayurvedic Constitution*, revised enlarged second edition, Sadhana Publications, Bellingham, WA 98225, 1998, good discussion of the dhatus, p. 73-89.

Tiwari, Maya, *Ayurveda: A Life of Balance*, simple, macrobiotic-style recipes for the doshas.

Programs:

Frawley, David, *Ayurvedic Healing Correspondence Course for Health Care Professionals*, Santa Fe, 1996, American Institute of Vedic Studies, PO Box 8357, Santa Fe, NM, 87504-8357, phone: (505) 983-9385, fax: (505) 982-5807, www.vedanet.com, email: vedicinst@aol.com. This course provides a thorough grounding in the basics of Ayurvedic healing, including in-depth information on the dhatus.

Women, Children, and Pregnancy:
BOOKS:

Blum, Jeanne Elizabeth, *Woman Heal Thyself: An Ancient Healing System for Contemporary Women*, a traditional Chinese medicine approach to the "forbidden points" related to menstruation, miscarriage, and pregnancy.

Peterson, Gayle, *Birthing Normally: A Personal Growth Approach to Childbirth*, second edition. This is a holistic approach from an unorthodox childbirth educator with rare skills. Working with visualization and counseling, she has helped many women, and couples, reframe current and past trauma in pregnancy in a workable and loving process.

Weed, Susun, *Wise Woman Herbal for the Childbearing Year*, lovely practical herbal focusing on pregnancy and lactation.

BUILDING HOME REMEDIES FROM DR. STONE: 1

BODY SYSTEM & Condition	HOME REMEDY:	OTHER RECOMMENDATIONS FROM STONE ON THIS CONDITION:
BLOOD **Anemia**	Fresh carrot, dandelion, parsley, spinach, and beet juice.	(1)
BLOOD VESSELS **Capillaries, weak or hemorrhaging**	Sesame seeds.	Grind the seeds and mix with water and "a little honey", daily. (2)
BONES AND JOINTS **Restoring natural curvature of the upper spine**	If you can comfortably (ed.), squat, with head bent gently forward.	One-half minute daily. (3)
Keeping joints and feet flexible	"Rub them (externally) with equal parts of oil and lemon juice." (4)	If you eat yogurt, use it only freshly made (24 hours or less after completion) and in small quantities. Ideally, an Indian-style lassi made with fresh yogurt diluted 1 to 4 with pure water is good. (5)
GASTRO-INTESTINAL TRACT **Digestive fire, low**	Small amounts of fresh ginger juice, taken with meals as needed.	Regular squatting strengthens digestive function. (6) Work "digestive" line on left thumb; see Chart #17 in chap. 6. Ed. note: see also METALS IN HEALING chart recommendations.
Ulcers, gastric & duodenal	Fresh carrot & cabbage juice, daily.	Also: sesame seed drink, see BLOOD VESSELS. (7)

BUILDING HOME REMEDIES FROM DR. STONE: 2

BODY SYSTEM & Condition	HOME REMEDY:	OTHER RECOMMENDATIONS FROM STONE ON THIS CONDITION:
HEART & CIRCULATION Poor circulation, heart needs to strengthen	Fresh carrot and beet juice. *	Work fleshy part of the thumb along lines referring to heart and cardiac muscles, see chart # 17, chapter 6.
Weak heart, recovery and rebuilding	Moderate action and the release of gases. Overall strategy: "When the diaphragm is free, the heart is free to act without fear or apprehension." (8) 1) Avoid fats, sweets, cholesterol, excess mineral oil, fried foods, over-heated animal fats. 2) Gentle rocking squats, when ready.	See ref. (9) Complete rest is needed in the acute stage, then the aim is to "help the heart patient to bring him (sic) back to as near a normal balance as Nature will permit." 1) Gently work the space between your thumb and forefinger on each hand. Also, work the cardiac and heart muscle reflexes on the fleshy part of the hand, see chart # 17, chap. 6. 2) Work on the feet: especially focus on the first joint of the second toe (the air toe, next to the big toe) on both feet. Work top to bottom and on either side of the toe, with a side-to-side motion. 3) Be sure you can breathe freely through both nostrils, especially the left one. 4) Craniosacral work can be valuable.(10)

BUILDING HOME REMEDIES FROM DR. STONE: 3

BODY SYSTEM & Condition	HOME REMEDY:	OTHER RECOMMENDATIONS FROM STONE ON THIS CONDITION:
NERVOUS SYSTEM **Anxiety and nervousness**	Let yourself keep moving freely: in swivel chairs, movable seats, rockers, swings, even rocking horses! (11)	1) side-to-side HA stretch (12) see chap. 2 in energizing stretch series 2) Yawning, sighing, deep breathing. *"Many a person groans himself into well-being..."* (13) 3) Relaxation posture: sit on floor with legs crossed, hands crossed, resting on knees. Breathe! (14)
Epilepsy	Fresh celery, carrot & lettuce juice.	8 oz. three or more times per day.
Nervous exhaustion	Same as above for epilepsy.	1) Evening meal of fresh fruit and warm milk. (15) 2) Reduce stress to nervous system, sympathetic nervous system especially.

BUILDING HOME REMEDIES FROM DR. STONE: 4

BODY SYSTEM & Condition	HOME REMEDY:	OTHER RECOMMENDATIONS FROM STONE ON THIS CONDITION:
NERVOUS SYSTEM (cont.) Sciatica	Overall strategy: improve digestion, reduce gas.	1) Hot packs to area. 2) Acute: BE CAREFUL! An adjustment could cause spasm. Instead, lie across bed or massage table width-wise, with your face down, to gently stretch. Use a pillow under your abdomen if that feels more comfortable. 3) If you can, gently & persistently work any sore points along your Achilles tendon, from ankle to mid-calf. 4) Feel for sore spots on the big toes, work them. Toe pulls can be helpful here. (16)
THYROID Goiter	A combination of fresh carrot & watercress* juice.	Ed. note: for specific Polarity bodywork recommendations that can be done with another person, see (17).
URINARY TRACT Kidney weak or inactive	Squats with motion. (18)	Work on kidney reflexes on outside of heel; see Chart # 17, chapter 6.

* "The juices of beets, parsley and watercress are very concentrated and should not be used too freely. About four ounces per day, mixed with other juices, is plenty." (19)

VIII.
———•———

CREATIVE ACTION

Rajas. Integrating Spirit, Mind and Body.
Pulse.

*"Opinions, thoughts, ideas, ideals are as real factors in
life as the food we eat."*
STONE, *POLARITY THERAPY, VOL. I, BK. 3, P. 13*

"Tuning in with the Infinite is a practical idea. . ."
STONE, *HEALTH BUILDING, P. 26*

RAJAS: SO WHAT ARE YOU GOING TO DO?

It is now mid-afternoon, moving toward evening in our
day together. These can be times of day when we stop and
question, need support, rest, or a nourishing pause. In the
larger scheme of things, it is a good time for creative action,
and sometimes a re-orientation.

In both Ayurveda and Polarity Therapy, healing is a
process that extends beyond the physical body to the heart,
mind and soul. While not every single practitioner of these
two healing arts is able to stretch skillfully in all these directions at all times, the systems themselves see each of these
dimensions as part of the whole. Both systems offer permission and support for balancing more than just the physical.

Practically, if we are attuned with our life purpose and
happy in what we are doing, life is likely to feel more joyous
and worthwhile. It is easier to deal with the physical, mental and emotional challenges that inevitably come along.
And conversely, when we are healthy and balanced in the
mental, emotional and physical realms, our life purpose may
be more readily achievable for us. This practical step-down

of energy is explored further in the questions which close this chapter; they are really what this chapter is all about.

To go further, when we are tense, worried, angry, or depressed, some muscles tighten, others slacken. Circulation is inhibited to some organs and enhanced to others. Our thoughts and feelings have a demonstrable effect on our physical bodies. Most of us have experienced this directly in one form or another, such as tight neck and shoulder muscles or an aching jaw in times of stress. For others of us, our back tightens, or hips, or an elbow. We express our feelings through our physical selves in patterns of movement, often unconsciously. We may not be aware of our thoughts or feelings, and yet our bodies are experiencing them.

Stone traced the effect of feelings to the energy currents. He noticed that when there was a block in feeling, there were corresponding blockages somewhere in the currents of the body. Because the free flow of energy was his intention for healing, he was interested in establishing a freer flow of feeling as well.

Similarly in Ayurveda, the doshas are seen as manifestations not only of physical biological energy, but also of emotion and mind. When we worry, Vata can accumulate in excess. And conversely, when Vata gets high, we may feel unaccountably worried or fearful. (Similarly, Pitta with anger and frustration, and Kapha with inertia or a desire to not move or be seen.) When the doshas get out of balance, we unconsciously respond to try to bring them back into balance. For example, if Vata or Pitta get too high, a lot of energy can move in an upward direction. We may not notice this consciously, and yet our bodies may shift their behaviors to adjust. Sometimes these adjustments are healthy ones, like slowing down and grounding more. Other times we may try to ground in other ways which ultimately frustrate us further, such as overeating.

Bringing an awareness that body, mind, feeling, and spirit all interrelate as one whole can be indispensable for healing. If we are not aware of our feelings, or mental agenda, or life purpose, or we ignore our body's needs, balance is harder to achieve. And yet awareness alone must be activated with something more. As one astute Polarity Therapist in training once said, " I think I have a pretty good idea of what I need to do. But... often I don't do it. Do you have any suggestions?"Awareness coupled with creative action and a relaxed acceptance of "what is" are keys here. Lest this sound impossibly difficult, I want to introduce specific techniques in this chapter that can help us do just this.

This dance to integrate what sometimes seem like very disparate energies can be challenging. Our bodies may pull us in one direction, our minds another, our souls yet a third way. It is this third way which gives life its deepest meaning, and yet we have responsibilities to our minds and bodies as well. I was fortunate to be able to study with a respected kahuna teacher, Morrnah Simeona, many years ago. She called the mind the mother of the body, and the body she considered the child. Our soul or spirit self she called the father self. One of her points was, it is important not to abandon the child, the body, while we are here living in it. (1)

How can we nurture our physicality and simultaneously pursue spiritual and mental goals? To paraphrase St. Francis of Assisi, we will not journey far without the help of Brother Ass (the body). If we can treat our bodies as manifestations of the divine, as a rare dance of male and female energies within, we are on track. Yet it is too easy to treat our physical selves just as we were treated as we grew up, with the same habits of indifference, excessive attention, or neglect. To break through the old into new patterns that meet current conditions more effectively is our challenge and aim.

What follows are a number of techniques that I have found effective over the past twelve years as an educator and counselor for re-aligning the larger energies of body, mind, and spirit. They are no substitute for a complete school of psychotherapy, such as Hakomi, transformational counseling, or psychosynthesis, any of which work very well with Polarity Therapy, and possibly with Ayurveda. Yet they are a beginning. To my knowledge, a full-blown educational curriculum of Ayurvedic and Polarity counseling does not yet exist; they are developments in process. Consequently, in this chapter I am simply offering an opening on how Polarity and Ayurveda might be used in this way, to get us started.

We will begin with a physical technique, go on to two mental-emotional processes, then explore a spiritual perspective. We will then circle back into an integration of these with the physical again, using movement and astrology in healing. Usually I would recommend doing one of these processes at a time; they are complete in and of themselves.

THE PULSE:

The first process works with the pulse, a core orientation point in Ayurvedic healing. This particular pulse technique comes from Polarity Therapy, however. It is quite easy to follow, even for a beginner. We start with the physical pulse.

There are many ways to read a pulse, and this is a simple straightforward one that you are likely to be able to do easily on yourself. Feel your wrist pulses, first one side and then the other. Is one side stronger than the other? Or are they about the same? This is the first point you are assessing. It gives you a beginning point for how to get yourself back in balance, if you are feeling "off".

If the left pulse is stronger than the right, this is a basic picture of over-extension. You are putting out more than your physical body can continue to sustain. If the reverse is true, that the right pulse is stronger than the left, you are holding energy back deep inside. This suppressing of energy can be as exhausting as any over-extending pattern.

What if neither of these patterns is true for you, and your pulses feel about equal in strength? Then you look at the relative strength of both pulses together. If both pulses are equally weak, you are likely to be tired, and needing rest and rejuvenation. The weaker the pulses, the more rest and healing you need. If both pulses are quite strong, more energy is available to you overall. It's important to note these are relative differences. The more difference there is between the two sides, the stronger the need for re-balancing. Sometimes the differences are almost negligible, and the need for change is minor. Feeling your own pulse gives tangible guidance on how you could support yourself more effectively. This can help build confidence in the appropriateness of a plan for healing.

This is one very simple beginning way to approach pulse. A skilled Ayurvedic or traditional Chinese medical practitioner would observe much more. And yet for our purposes, there is plenty to be learned in working with just this much.

If the left pulse is stronger, the energy is extended out to your periphery, and your aim is to bring some of it back into your core. You have been sending out a lot of energy (in a centrifugal way), and it is time to invite it back in (in a centripetal approach). Generally the blockages in this situation relate to receiving, allowing energy in. Physically working with your gut can start to bring this energy back into alignment. At the same time it is important to assess your lifestyle, and ask yourself where you could be over-extending. What are you willing to cut out? Or perhaps it is not so much a matter of physically over-doing it as mentally or emotionally over-extending. This attitude is also reflected in this kind of pulse. For example, it can be revealed in an approach which values taking care of others more than oneself. Or the basic workaholic approach of "I'll just finish this one last thing before I eat," even though you are hungry now. It is also the kind of pulse associated with an over-expenditure of emotional energy. Some suggestions on how to work further with this pulse are offered in the table that follows. When the left pulse is stronger, it is of benefit to support and strengthen the parasympathetic nervous system.

When the right pulse is noticeably stronger, more energy is being held in the spine and the core, from a Polarity perspective. Here you have been taking in energy and ideas (in a centripetal way), and it is time to send energy back out (with centrifugal action). Usually the majority of blockages in this situation relate to putting out energy; for example, creative energy. In this case, physically supporting and relaxing your back is where you begin. In working on the back, you are inviting the energy to relax and be released from your core. Heat to the spine, in the form of hot showers or packs, helps release stagnant circulation there physically. Yoga, movement and bodywork are excellent supports here. Are there creative projects you would like to share with the world that you haven't yet done? Do ideas about community service come to you, hopes and dreams of projects you hope to achieve in your life? Now is the time to begin to bring them into manifestation. There is accumulated energy within you that would appreciate being expressed. Look at where you may be holding back to give yourself clues as to where you need to balance this energy. The expression "waiting to exhale" is a perfect description of the right-dominant pulse. It's okay to take in a breath, and let it out: exhale completely. The over-worked sympathetic nervous system is what needs initial support.

The beauty of the pulse is that it is a reliable indicator of your current condition. You don't have to guess about your relative balance, you can immediately feel it in your pulses. The pulses do not lie, although medications can affect them in a variety of ways. Your pulse lets you know how your body and psyche are responding to the life you have created. Each person is different in how much activity they can handle and how much stimulation they need. Your pulse gives you an answer as to where you stand now, and how you can best move into greater balance.

The pulse has been used for centuries as an assessment tool in healing. Both Ayurveda and traditional Chinese medicine have subtle and detailed methods of reading the pulse, which can take decades to master. This is a simple, easy, uncomplicated approach directly from Dr. Stone that can give you a good first estimate of how you can best work with yourself. In his writings Randolph Stone primarily referred to it as a way to balance physical conditions. Feel free to consult a skilled practitioner of pulse for further insights.

The best time to get a fair sense of the pulse is on an empty stomach, and not immediately after intense exercise or a bath or shower.

PULSES: LEFT-RIGHT DIFFERENCES

Pulse:	Implies:	Begin work with:	Specifics:
right pulse stronger	energy held in the "core": in the spine and back	The back. Exhalation. Applying more centrifugal approaches in your life.	Yoga for the back. Hot showers, especially along your spine. Back rubs. Visualize extending your resources out into the world.
left pulse stronger	energy extended out to the periphery of the body	The gut. Inhalation. Applying more centripetal approaches in your life; it's okay to receive.	Massage & yoga for the abdomen. Movement that tones the abdominal muscles. Hot packs to the belly. Cold showers to the spine. Imagine drawing your resources back home to your core; see A PRACTICE OF COMING INTO STILLNESS, chapter 4.

PULSES: LEFT-RIGHT DIFFERENCES (cont.)

Pulse:	Implies:	Begin work with:	Specifics:
right & left are about the same and strong	resources are balanced	Either centrifugal or centripetal actions, maintaining a balance.	A balance of front and back, outer and inner activities.
right & left are about the same, yet weak on both sides	resources are low in the body as a whole	Rest. Rebuilding energy.	Address any specific illnesses. Schedule regular times for rest. Begin to create realistic limits based on how much energy you expend.

(2)

CENTRIFUGAL AND CENTRIPETAL: A REVIEW

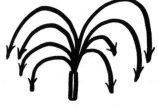

Centrifugal

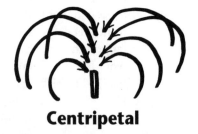

Centripetal

"Life must ever flow as a fountain from within out, and we call the return currents the experience of life." (3)

CENTRIFUGAL	**CENTRIPETAL**
Create, expand.	**Relax, receive.**
Exhale.	**Inhale.**
Go out.	**Return.**
Light, day.	**Darkness, night.**

There are many ways to integrate this information into every day life. For example, you might take more time to breathe out, if you have a stronger right pulse. For those of us with strong left pulses, longer inhales can be the experiment. For example, these differences in breath can be incorporated into the Polarity Yoga stretches presented in chapter 2. Do the movements as presented. Yet, if your right pulse is hardier, give yourself more time to exhale, and as you do, imagine you are releasing that which you are holding inside. If it is the left pulse which is the robust one, focus your attention on the inhale, and allowing energy to come to you.

In Viniyoga, breath is used to build or cleanse. If you inhale as you move into a challenging stretch, this is building to that area. If you exhale as you take on the stretch, this cleanses the area. Gary Kraftsow in *Yoga for Wellness* incorporates many of these concepts in quite skillful ways. For example, posture #5 in the POLARITY YOGA TO RELAX routine in chapter 2 can be done as a traditional yoga asana, Supta Baddha Konasana. Kraftsow combines breath and mantra in this position to ease premenstrual pain or menopausal congestion. To explain a little further how to do this, he uses the mantra, OH MA OH, honoring the Divine Mother in many traditions. You begin with the stretch shown in chapter 2, knees open, soles of the feet touching. Instead of holding this stretch on the floor as we did in chapter 2, you bring your knees up 1/3 of the way while you exhale, chanting OH MA OH. When you have finished exhaling, you hold that position 1/3 of the way up and inhale. Then you bring your knees another 1/3 of the way to close, exhaling with OH MA OH. And so forth, until your knees are together, pointing toward the ceiling. Usually it would be repeated about six times. The specific intention of the exercise is to improve circulation in the perineal floor. The focus on exhale would be helpful for cleansing the pelvic area of tension, and could also assist right-robust pulse types. Clearly this is one posture taken out of context; it is given as part of a short program for PMS in *Yoga for Wellness*. (4) And yet it could give the more exploratory among us encouragement to adventure beyond the confines of what has been presented here. There are many ways to bring ourselves and our pulses into balance.

THE GUNAS IN LIFE

All three gunas manifest in every experience, as Randolph Stone emphasized. One friend of mine, a Polarity Therapist, learned this in a vivid way. He was invited to join a group Polarity practice, sharing offices with other therapists in a cooperative venture. He vigorously declined the initial invitation, because he thought his individual practice was working well for him. Soon after, he had a dream that put the group practice in a very favorable light. He awoke, strongly attracted to the idea of joining the cooperative practice. He called back his colleagues. The situation had changed. They said they needed time to sort out whether his participation was still possible. My friend fell into a funk. The more time passed, the more convinced he became that the group practice was for him. And the longer he waited for a call, the more thoughts of worthlessness began to haunt him. He even began to think that without the group practice, he was nothing: a 180 degree shift from his original position!

Being a perceptive individual, he sat down with himself and noticed a few things. He had acted strongly, declining the invitation (action=rajas). He had then become deeply attached to the idea (attraction=tamas). He realized he'd gotten stuck between these two gunas. How so? He wasn't sure. He decided, why not ask to experience sattva, the third guna, here? What would it be like to experience this situation in a sattvic way? Over the course of this day, surprising thoughts came to him. He found himself remembering his grandfather, who had grown up in the Depression. He remembered his grandfather saying how hard it was to find work then, and how he had had to work alone. His grandfather had said this with some chagrin, as if working alone was not as good as being able to work with others.

My friend began to wonder if his feelings were even his own, or if perhaps he had fallen into old family patterns of thinking. As he realized this, a thought popped spontaneously into his mind, "I have always been worthy." Surprised at this thought, he found himself relaxing; it felt true. With this thought central in his experience, he realized that whether the new group practice welcomed him or he continued in his individual practice, each was okay with him.

Here clear, neutral sattva offered him healing. Yet there are other times when rajas or tamas will do the same. When we need to act on something, it is rajas that mobilizes us. When we need to commit to something, become attached and complete a process, tamas assists us.

THE GUNAS IN LIFE: A PROCESS

You can play with looking at a current situation in your own life with the following inquiries, or similar ones. Think of the situation with which you would like to work. Give yourself a few quiet moments to reflect on the situation. When you are ready, ask to:

Experience tamas in this situation. What attracts you here? To what are you attached?

Let yourself experience rajas in this situation. What has your action been in this situation? Are there any actions you want to take?

Let yourself experience sattva. If you were going to speak from within your neutral core (sattva), what words come to you about this situation?

Generally, tamas will come forward as some kind of attachment, rajas as an action or desire for action, and sattva will be unconditional in nature, like the statement that came to my friend in the story above.

MEDIATION AND YOUR MIND-BODY RELATIONSHIP:

This next process is a more mentally-oriented approach, a mind-body mediation for times of inner conflict. (Illness and fatigue, for example, qualify as potential imbalances and conflicts.) The pulse gives us one orientation to our body's condition; and the gunas process gives us one picture of how we are using their energies. The mind-body mediation gives us a chance to check in on this relationship more specifically.

If you are facing a challenge, either physical, emotional or mental, which has been persistent or seems insurmountable, the following process can be illuminating. It works especially well if you are accustomed to meditation, visualization, or any kind of inner dialoguing.

MIND-BODY MEDIATION:

Relax and let yourself get comfortable. Any restful position is fine. A notebook and pen close by may come in handy. You are going to be asking yourself a few questions. Before you do, here's a brief explanation of what you're about to do.

In any illness (dis-ease), there is usually a conflict of some sort: between the immune system and the germs, or the part that wants to be well and the part that is sick, or the part of us that is tired and the part that is restless, to give a few possibilities. Often we are well aware of one part, and may be giving another side short shrift. This process is based on two concepts:

* we are potential mediators of our own conflicts, and

* we can access the resources of both our body and our mind.

It is important to realize here that the mind and body are actually a continuum, rather than two distinct and separate energies. Yet, given the age in which we live, often you will find that body and mind have been compartmentalized in their roles, into two separate rooms of all that is you. This process invites them into the same "room" and hopefully gets them dialoguing with one another again.

So you relax, take a few deep breaths, and ask the following questions:

1) Body, what do you need?

Sit and wait until you get some sort of answer. It may be a picture, or feelings, or words, or a sensation. If you like, jot the response down.

2) Mind, can you imagine a positive outcome to our dilemna or challenge?

Same procedure.

3) Body and mind, are you willing to work together?

Again, wait for a response. If the answer is yes, go on to the last question.

4) How would you like to work together?

The first time this process occurred to me, I was away from home on a retreat, with a wracking cough. Earlier that day, a new friend Zach Burney had demonstrated a powerful healing potential of the mind, asking the mind to help the body stretch beyond its accustomed limits. I was impressed with how well his method worked with the mind, and I was inspired to include the body in the equation as well. While I'd dosed myself with rest, and vitamin C, and garlic, and various supportive herbs, I hadn't really stopped to ask both my body and mind: "Hey, what's going on for you here? How can I help now?"

The cough was a nasty one. In checking in, I realized my mind had far more optimism about healing this bug than I had been aware. It suggested a specific cleansing meditation and chant that felt instinctively right for me. My body said that it missed my partner's comforting touch; touch was what my body needed more than anything else at that moment. I put my hands on my chest and it did feel comforting. Both my mind and body said they were willing to work together to heal this situation. The cough did not go away immediately, but my hand on my chest calmed its wracking quality to something I could sleep with easily, a welcome shift.

Since that time, I have shared these questions with a number of people, with hopeful results. What I have also noticed so far, with some surprise, is that in some long-standing apparently physical illnesses, it has been the mind in the feuding parties that refuses to cooperate. That is, the body has a healing answer, the mind has a healing answer, and then both are asked if they are willing to work together. Invariably so far in my experiences with others, the body is willing to cooperate, but the mind is not always ready. (5) (6) This leads me to offer the following process, for those times when our mind or emotions are balking, and yet we really don't understand why. This drawing process invites us to open beyond mind to our larger self.

LETTING EMOTIONAL ENERGY BE AND MOVE:

Dr. Stone wrote, "*In the emotional field* (pain) *also rests on the face of an un-assimilated sensation.*" (7) The focus of the following process is to acknowledge the pain or discomfort of an area, whether it be physical, emotional, or spiritual, and begin to let it assimilate back into the energy flow of the body. This third process works more with our spiritual selves in a drawing process based on Tibetan psychology, though it can also be used to deal with feelings or physical issues.

DRAWING PROCESS BASED ON TIBETAN PSYCHOLOGY

You will be doing this with a series of drawings. It can be quite fun, especially if you have colors you like. Oil pastels or crayons work well, on recycled newsprint. The size of the paper does not matter too much, just let it be big enough that you can draw quickly, without constriction. You will need four whole pieces of paper, and probably about a half hour's length of time.

The specific sequence of drawings you are about to do can be used to move energy, or simply to get clearer about what might be going on for you, in the larger picture, so to speak. You can also apply it to specific problems or challenges, any condition which holds a feeling for you. It is based on concepts used in Tibetan Buddhist psychology; the process developed for me when I was training in a Master's program in counseling using art in the mid 1980's.

In my preliminary learning about Tibetan Buddhist psychology, I understood that in this system, every feeling is acknowledged. The view is that every feeling has a function and that each emotion does something for us. There was not a strong judgment about feelings being good or bad, they all have their place. This was the original perspective. (8) This particular approach holds a fair amount in common with Tibetan Dzog-Chen, which invites us to open to "what is", regardless of what it is. (9)

In Tibetan Buddhist psychology, the same feeling, such as anger, may have one function for one person and a completely different function for another. For example, when Lisa gets mad, she goes off and is by herself. Her anger gives her space (whether she wants it or not is another matter). Her friend Michael gets mad, and hollers at other drivers on the road. The way he uses anger expresses his fire, gets it out. His friend Jennifer gets mad, and wants to have a fight. Her anger's function is to get her more connected with the people she loves, to be passionately involved. Now, again, whether any of these strategies work or feel comfortable, is a whole other story.

Feelings are mysterious and multi-dimensional, so whatever emotion you are experiencing just now, may have different roots or effects than you consciously imagine. The following process invites you to begin to navigate this mysterious territory with a boat and paddle. You will be working quickly and trusting your first impulses. There is no need to try to figure it out. In fact, the less you think during these processes, the better.

You will have four drawings on four pieces of paper. For many of us, especially these days with trees being cleared from the forests so very fast, there is an urge to save paper and draw on both sides of two sheets. You need four sheets so that when you're done, you can see the whole sequence at once. I like to use recycled newsprint, and recycle it again, if I can. Whatever. Colors in hand, let yourself get quiet and answer each question by drawing.

Drawing #1: *What's the feeling you want to work with now?*

This can be an uncomfortable or comfortable feeling or a sensation, whatever you want to work with.

Simply draw the feeling on which you are focussing, let it come out however it would like.

Drawing #2: *What's the function of the feeling?*

Ask yourself, how is this feeling serving me right now? What is this feeling doing for me? Let yourself draw the answer, as best you can. Now is not the time to get caught up in self-analysis. Just draw the function of the feeling, let your hand do it, not your brain.

Drawing #3: *What is the hidden treasure of the feeling?*

This is tricky, because this is what you don't know about the feeling. Relax, get quiet inside and let your hand answer this question: what is the hidden treasure of this feeling?

Drawing #4: *What now?*

You follow the same process here: don't think, just draw. The question is: what now?

When you're finished, spread all four drawings in front of you; let yourself look at them. How do you feel?

You may find the drawings have titles. Feel free to title them. Or you can label them: *1: Feeling, 2: Function of the Feeling, 3: Hidden Treasure,* and *4: What Now?* You may think you don't care about the date, but if you're at all inclined, it's helpful to put dates on the back and consider saving them. Later, they may be a telling comment on this period of your life. Or you can toss them immediately. The point is to let them do their work. And what they are here for is to help you move stuck energy. First you see it, then you acknowledge its function, then you acknowledge its treasure, then you let the next step emerge. (10)

You may want some idea about the kind of issues that respond well to this kind of process. I've seen people use it with relief in depression, pain, attraction, resistance (say to a diet or self-care plan), pregnancy, dying, abuse, the unknown.

The first three drawings get energy moving and help identify consciously what may be going on. The last drawing elicits commitment, to something, often some kind of change. And yet, the rub is, you don't know what the change or potential commitment will be until you've drawn it. Risky business!

WRITING:

A few people, maybe two in twenty, really don't enjoy drawing. Or maybe you just love to write. You can do the same process as above writing, in a journal. The thing about drawing is, it really draws out the right brain (pardon my pun) and its symbolic functions. So it's an especially good balance for those of us who ceaselessly analyze. What I'd say about drawing is, try it first, even if you think you won't like it. You can always journal later.

OTHER WAYS OF WORKING:

Each of these first three processes is complete in itself. Yet all three usually work in fairly quiet ways, primarily seated, for example. Sometimes movement is an essential ingredient for integration. A number of years ago, I was presenting how the drawing process above could be used to deal with emotional hunger to a Polarity Therapy class. One Polarity Therapist in training, Mary, listened intently. She took one look at me, and said emphatically, "That would never work for me. When that kind of feeling or sensation arises, I need to move. " The certainty with which she said it spoke its truth. She went on to say that thinking about it as I described would not help her at all. She knew this sensation well. And for her, she knew just how to deal with it: intense physical movement. She knew that in this situation for her, an intensely rajasic response was the healthy one. And this is true for many people.

Astrology combined with movement can integrate the conscious and the unconscious in ways different than those so far presented.

MOVEMENT AND ASTROLOGY:

Dr. Stone was an adventurous character; he did not balk at exploring the esoteric. Among his adventures, he used Western astrology and the four elements to design yoga exercises. (11) In Western medicinal astrology, each of the astrological signs of Aries through Pisces relate to a part of the body. Dr. Stone created yoga stretches with this and the elements in mind. For example, in his squatting postures, he consciously lined up the three areas of the body that relate to air, or what he called the "Airy Triad". (12) In his experience, gently easing oneself down into a squat harmonized the flow of air and prana in many ways, specifically relieving the body of gas and worry. (Or what an Ayurvedic practitioner would call calming Vata.)

The embryo (fetus) in the mother's womb, woven by the energy lines of the four elements in their three-fold action.

CHART NO. 5

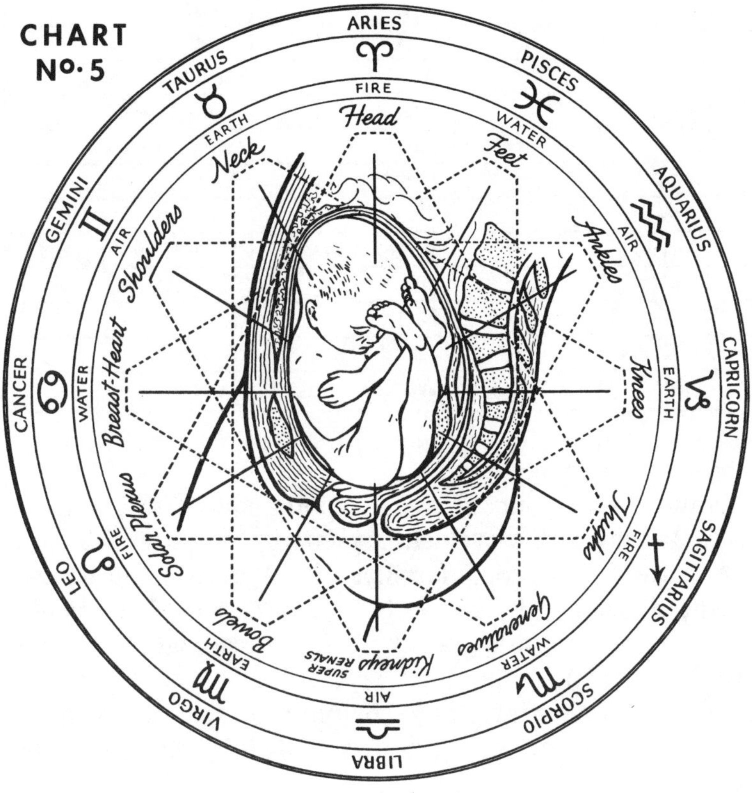

(13)

"The position of the child in the mother's womb is the natural squatting posture of man, where all energy currents can flow freely to produce a perfect human body, and for maintaining good health after birth and throughout life in this world. (Please refer to my book, *"Easy Stretching Postures for Vitality and Beauty"*. This is the origin of it and here is the reason for its fine results as a NATURAL HEALTH EXERCISE.)"

Chart #5: Embryo in the Mother's Womb. Reprinted from Dr. Randolph Stone, *Polarity Therapy*, vol. I, bk. 1, p. 49, with gracious permission by CRCS Publications.

MOVING THROUGH THE ZODIAC

Astrological Sign	Element	Body zone
Aries	Fire	Head
Taurus	Earth	Neck
Gemini	Air	Shoulders
Cancer	Water	Breast-heart
Leo	Fire	Solar plexus
Virgo	Earth	Bowels
Libra	Air	Kidneys-adrenals
Scorpio	Water	Generative organs
Sagittarius	Fire	Thighs
Capricorn	Earth	Knees
Aquarius	Air	Ankles
Pisces	Water	Feet

(14)

Simply using your Sun sign as a point of departure, you can begin to play with movement and energy blockages in a more focused way. For people familiar with Ayurveda and Jyotish, (Vedic astrology), I want to be clear that in this particular process, we are working with Western astrology. And yet it would be easy enough, and fascinating, I would guess, to apply the same principles to the more complex workings of the nakshatras and planets as they relate in a Vedic chart. (15)

Here we will be working with the sun. In Western astrology, the sun relates to our essential self, our core. You will be inviting forward your deepest sense of who you are as you move. Let yourself orient with your spine, breathe in and out through your spine. When you feel centered here, move your awareness to the part of your body related to your sun sign (see MOVING THROUGH THE ZODIAC table). For example, if you are an Aries sun sign, it would be your head, as a Taurus, your focus would be your neck, and so on. Begin to initiate your movements from this one area. If you move your hand, let the movement come first from the area related to your sun. Center all your movements around this part of your body. If you wish to couple this with a question, you can begin to ask, "Who am I?" as you move. Move as long as you like, trusting the movement which arises. When you feel complete, stop and come back to breathing through your spine.

If you like, you can jot down reflections on this process. As you moved, did a different area than the one you intended try to lead movements? Which areas tended to hold back? Was there anywhere in your body you felt stuck? If you wanted to pursue these areas further you could, either from an elemental triad approach or through work with the currents that flow over them.

The entire horoscope can be danced in this way, weaving in relationships between the planets, signs and houses. For more information about this, see the appendix, MORE ABOUT ASTROLOGY AND MOVEMENT.

ABOUT SEXUAL ENERGY:

Part of our creative energy is our sexual energy. Polarity Therapy and Ayurveda together hold potential keys to clearer more joyous sexuality. Physically and energetically, there are places you can begin to orient here. These include: assessing your right-left pulses: does energy need to be drawn out from the core (right stronger) or invited back into the core (left stronger)? Where are the safe zones in your body, where you can safely connect with your own sensuous energies? (Sensuous: connecting with the senses, relationship: allowing yourself to connect with another). Each of us is different in how we connect with our own energies and those of someone else. It's okay to acknowledge and respect the places where you connect, and the places where you are different.

Sexuality is a subtle process of connection on many levels. Each of us plays with both the masculine and feminine within, to varying degrees. Biologically, men and women use different energies to procreate, which can give us clues to archetypal energies. That is, very simply, to create a child, a man must get seed out, move outward, expand. A woman takes this seed inward, receives and nurtures it. Hers is a conservative protective act, in order to successfully conceive, while his is an outgoing one. Clearly within any mutually consenting sensuous connection, all three principles of life come into play. We are simultaneously expansive, contractive, giving, receiving, neutral. How comfortable with each of these roles we are, can be our edge for growth and joy.

The dance between masculine and feminine energies is evident in any relationship. In my work with same gender couples, there is definitely an interplay of both masculine and feminine, regardless of the gender of the couple.

Trust is a crucial part of any intimate relationship. The levels of trust run back to our earliest infancy, probably even to conception. How much we trust ourselves and our partner sets many of the parameters for how deeply we can explore with one another. Sometimes it is not the person we mistrust, but their gender, based on our past experiences. Many of us have had experiences in our lives that have led us not to trust. Trust is something that can be built slowly, with safe boundaries. It is okay to be patient with yourself on this. As someone I respect said candidly about his marriage, "When I found I could trust (my wife), it was very important. I haven't trusted women deeply. In trusting my wife, I found I could begin to trust my own maleness." For him, trusting one sex allowed him to begin to trust his own sex. And yet this was no overnight process, much as we sometimes wish intimacy could be.

Letting go of expectation can really help free up a relationship, though again, it can be easier said than done. Physical expectations can be deeply inhibiting: one woman and man I know almost sunk their sexual relationship in the serious job of conceiving a child. Other couples have struggles related to strong ideas about what their specific sexual needs are. It is important to meet one another where we are. If we are genuinely interested in connecting, we will; though perhaps not always in the way we have in mind. Healthy relationships also include deep interpersonal connections of a sexual nature which can be nourishing, and yet non-genital.

Polarity Therapy's focus of freeing up blockages in energy can be a true ally in healthy sexual exploration. If you wish to connect more deeply with your own sexuality, inviting energy down into the spiral current or long lines can be very potent. When you are coming into your own identity vis-a-vis your sexual expression, work with the transverse current can make the most sense (see chapter 2 for more information about the currents). On a physical level, combining the rejuvenative effects of Ayurvedic medicated ghee (see appendix PERSONAL CARE recipes) with Dr. Stone's time-honored openness to being with the perineum, can be profoundly satisfying and nurturing, whether you are massaging yourself or a loved one. Working up and down the spine with love, respect and rejuvenative ghee can feel quite wonderful.

From the perspective of Western nutrition, when we are deficient in nutrients, particularly vitamin E and zinc, our libido literally deflates. These nutrients are essential to a healthy sexual drive for both sexes.

CHAPTER SYNOPSIS:

CREATIVE ACTION:

POLARITY: THE STEP-DOWN OF ENERGY IN FORM:

Are you expressing your life purpose fully and creatively?

Can you understand what it is
you came here in this life to be and do?

Can you hold with yourself in a neutral way
as you get ready to receive the support
you need to fulfill this purpose?

Can you open to the breath of life,
receive what you need into your lungs and being?

Can you digest these experiences
and absorb them as fully as you need?

Are you willing to create new expressions of this purpose
and offer them to others?

Are you ready to let go of what you no longer need to
get on with this creative process of living?

RESOURCES IN CREATIVE ACTION:
BOOKS:

Alon, Ruthy, *Mindful Spontaneity*, includes a Feldenkrais look at sexuality as a creative and healthy process of movement, p. 145-170.

Chitty, John and Anna, *Relationships and the Human Energy Field: Training Course Manual*, Polarity Center of Colorado, Boulder, CO, 1991, primary effort in Polarity Therapy to date to integrate Polarity with modern counseling approaches, especially drawing on the work of Pia Mellody and others.

Mind in Buddhist Psychology, a translation of Ye-shes rgyal-mtshan's "The Necklace of Clear Understanding" by Herbert V. Guenther and Leslie S. Kawamura, Dharma Publishing, Emeryville, California, 1975. Delightfully open look at feelings, fairly densely written.

Perera, Sylvia Brinton, *Descent to the Goddess: A Way of Initiation for Women*, this Jungian classic encourages us to stand in our power and face our own darkness with beauty.

Stone, *Polarity Therapy*, vol. II, p. 209-213, about differences between the right and left pulse.

PROGRAMS:

Levine, Peter, PhD, Somatic Experiencing Workshops, offers a unique way to literally unwind trauma using simple questions and counseling techniques. Foundation for Human Enrichment, PO Box 1872, Lyons, CO, 80540, (303) 823-9524, ergos@earthlink.net. See also Levine, *Waking the Tiger*, especially the chapters 16 & 17, "Administering (Emotional) First Aid After An Accident" and "First Aid for Children", p. 235-264.

Self I-dentity through Ho'ponopono, The Foundation of I, Inc, PO Box 10861, Honolulu, HI 96816-0861, phone/fax: (808) 395-9278, based on the work of kahuna Morrnah Simeona.

See also the work of Lee Cartwright, listed in RESOURCES in chapter 2.

ASTROLOGY REFERENCES THAT DIRECTLY RELATE TO THIS CHAPTER:

Arroyo, Stephen, *Astrology, Psychology and the Four Elements: An Energy Approach to Astrology & Its Use in the Counseling Arts*, p. 79-86 and p. 157-170.

Greene, Liz, *Mythic Astrology*, a deck of introductory cards to begin to play with the concepts presented here.

Spiller, Jan, *Astrology for the Soul*, focuses on clarifying our higher purpose through understanding the north and south nodes of the moon in our Western natal chart.

IX.

———•———

HEALING

Opening to the Subtle Dimensions

"The infinite within is ever becoming."
STONE, *HEALTH BUILDING*, P. *164*

A good deal of information has been given here for self-healing; it's time to take stock and see how you can integrate it on your own behalf. At the end of this chapter you will find a self-care plan to fill out to focus your healing intentions. As we begin to complete our day together, there are some areas of experience from Polarity and Ayurveda that still need to be included to create a whole picture. For many centuries, healing has included subtle as well as more concrete methods for supporting health. We have already dealt with unseen energies in the form of the Ayurvedic doshas and Polarity currents, and seen their strong role in healing. In this chapter, we will be exploring further some of the more subtle or esoteric dimensions of healing.

THE KOSHAS:

Ayurveda and Yoga refer to protective energy sheaths around our bodies. These are known in Sanskrit as *koshas*, in their protective enclosing sense, or as *mayas*, when their function is to open our awareness and expand into universal consciousness. Kosha: protection. Maya: expanding consciousness. Collectively in Western parapsychology they are often called the aura. In metaphysics, they are sometimes referred to as "the three bodies", that is, the physical body, the astral body and the causal body. They have also been described as the five or six sheaths, depending on whether the physical body, the "food sheath", *annamaya kosha*, is included in the tally. All of these terms are describing the same thing: that is, our physical body and the entire energetic field surrounding it.

The Koshas

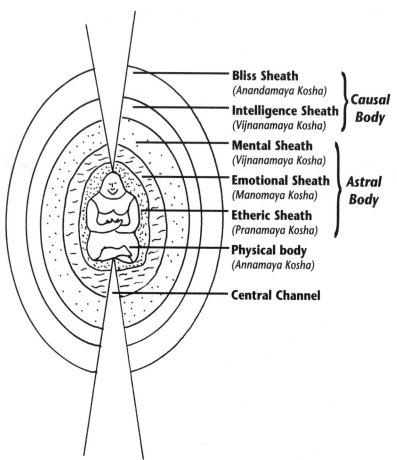

Bliss Sheath
(Anandamaya Kosha)
Intelligence Sheath
(Vijnanamaya Kosha)

Causal Body

Mental Sheath
(Vijnanamaya Kosha)
Emotional Sheath
(Manomaya Kosha)
Etheric Sheath
(Pranamaya Kosha)

Astral Body

Physical body
(Annamaya Kosha)

Central Channel

How the koshas and the currents relate is yet to be mapped in any extensive way. In my experience, the three energy currents of Polarity are like the "wireless anatomy" not only of our physical bodies, but also our energetic sheaths. Practically I mention this because many subtle energies can accumulate in the field around our bodies and can be released in the same ways, often as we release blockages in the physical. That is, patterns, habits, feelings, and beliefs are held not just in the musculature of the body, but also in the energy field around the body. These energetic accumulations can be contacted through breath work, meditation, movement, or subtle bodywork, with some points being contacted off the body, some on it.

From Randolph Stone's own description of the location of the long lines on the body, one would surmise that he first experienced them primarily in the second sheath, the pranamaya kosha. This energy body, also known as the etheric sheath, is located immediately off the physical body. In accord with their location, the long line currents' function is in part to clear and strengthen breath and energy (prana or chi). By working with the long lines in the pranamaya kosha, one helps create new blueprints of health there, which can then manifest in the physical body. Stone said the long lines could be found running both just off the body and within the musculature at its surface. (1)

The spiral current and transverse current can be less contained. In fact, each of the currents can expand and contract with variations in our personal accumulation of energy and the way the energy runs in these patterns. This inevitable flow of energy outward and back to the core relies on a return pathway in each current. We must be able to both put out energy, expand, in what Dr. Stone would call a centrifugal pattern of expansion and outward movement, and be able to bring energy back into the core, what he would call a receptive, inward, contracting, centripetal flow. This balance of putting out and taking in is at the foundation of a healthy life. (2) (3)

Just as congestion can build up in the physical body, congestion can arise in the energetic fields surrounding the physical body. For some people this may be easier to grasp than for others. To try to make it more tangible, here is an analogy from Earth. Many years ago, when the first pictures of our planet were taken from space, there was little clutter seen in the gravitational field around the earth. Yet in the ensuing thirty-some years of space exploration, we humans have introduced many objects, "space junk" into the earth's atmosphere, in the form of satellites and such. These continue to orbit about the earth, sometimes for decades, before they are decommissioned or disintegrate.

Similarly, energetic congestion can build up in the field just off our bodies, which has an impact on emotional and mental health as well as our physical well-being. This congestion, or what have been called skandas, patterns of accumulation in the Buddhist tradition, can be literally felt or seen by some people when contacting the field around the physical body. (4) Many indigenous traditions acknowledge this point with various sorts of cleansings of this field. Here in North America, smudgings with sage or copal are examples of this. The ritual cleansings with water undertaken by a Muslim or Sufi before prayer might also be said to fulfill the same function.

Right now I mention this primarily so you can be aware that when you are doing healing with yourself, whether in the form of singing, chanting, praying, dancing, or bodywork, it is likely you are working on your koshas as well as your physical body.

THE USE OF METALS IN HEALING:

As we are working with subtler energies, the energies of mind and breath, another subtle healer is metal. Metal has been used for many centuries in healing in a variety of ways. While in the East Indian system of Ayurveda specially potentized metals are sometimes taken internally as *bhasma* (ash) or *churnas* (powders), in Polarity Therapy silver and gold are used primarily externally. In Ayurveda, silver is considered a cooling energy, while gold is a warming one. In Polarity, too, silver is valued for its role as a cooling agent and gold for its ability to warm.

For Dr. Stone, *"Metals are living things."* (5) He was quite interested in this method of balancing the energy currents. He told the following story: *"The Hindus worship a trinity of gods whom they call Brahma, Vishnu and Shiva, much the same as Christians worship God the Father, God the Son and God the Holy Ghost. It is said that many thousands of years ago Vishnu gave to his followers and devotees the secret of healing by means of herbs, leaves and plants and the finer energies hidden in them. The followers of Shiva came to him and complained that they had to go to the followers of Vishnu to get relief from their ailments because they had received no such means from their own god, Shiva. Shiva replied: 'I will give you something much better; that is the secret of the energy latent in metals for use in healing yourselves. This is much more potent than the energy in the herbs and vegetables.' This knowledge served the people for a long, long time, until the secret was forgotten and the understanding of the principle was lost."* (6)

Included here are two tables compiled from Stone's recommendations about metals in healing, which you can peruse and experiment with on your own. These are formed from his unique perspective, which has some roots in the Vedic tradition, and yet diverges from it at times. Gemstones also offer excellent healing resources. This is not a formal part of Polarity Therapy, and yet it is a field that has been explored extensively in Jyotish, Vedic astrology, in support of Ayurvedic healing. In the RESOURCE section which follows, Drs. Lad and Bhattacharya have generously opened vistas into this knowledge of gems and healing in their respective books: Sree Chakravarti has done essential work with mudras and color for healing, described in her work, *A Healer's Journey*.

POLARITY: PLANETARY CORRESPONDENCES WITH METALS

PLANET:	*METALS:*
Sun	gold
Moon	silver
Mercury	mercury
Venus	copper and brass
Mars	iron
Jupiter	tin and zinc

(7)

THE USE OF METALS IN HEALING BY DR. STONE

BODY AREA OR SYSTEM	CONDITION	RECOMMENDATION
BONES AND JOINTS	Rheumatoid arthritis	1) Copper or zinc bracelet 2) Copper & zinc insoles in shoes to relieve pain
DIGESTIVE SYSTEM	Digestive fire low	Wear gold ring on (left) middle finger
	Hemorrhoids	Wear silver ring on little finger
HEART & CIRCULATION	Heart: sluggish	Gold ring on (left) forefinger (wear with caution: stimulating)
	Heart: over stimulated	Silver ring on (left) forefinger
MIND	Sluggish	Wear gold ring on (left) thumb, silver ring on (left) big toe
REPRODUCTIVE SYSTEM	Pelvic inflammation	Wear silver ring on fourth toe
	Sluggish, congested	Wear gold ring on fourth (ring) finger. (ed: Contra-indicated if any pelvic inflammation)
RESPIRATORY SYSTEM	Sluggish, congested	Wear gold ring on (left) forefinger
STAGNATION	In feet and legs	Stand on a silver plate!
TEETH	Neuralgia, acute	Press the painful tooth with a gold ring or object. Sun the tooth (or ring?) if possible
TEMPERATURE OF THE BODY	Too cold	Draw a gold comb lightly over the body
	Too hot	Draw a silver comb lightly over the body

(8)

POLARITY, HOMEOPATHY AND WESTERN MEDICINE:

Randolph Stone believed Polarity Therapy was an appropriate modality to use with just about any other method of healing. In particular he saw Polarity as a way to unite divergent practices, such as homeopathy and Western medicine. (9) He saw the flexibility of Polarity, in that it could work in an outgoing, expansive manner, (centrifugal) as does Western medicine, or it could be used to work in a receptive way (centripetal), as does homeopathy. Because Polarity energetically encompasses an understanding of how both systems work, and includes both expansive and contractive work in its philosophical base, it can be successfully used with either one.

Dr. Stone considered the centrifugal approach one of healing with opposites; the centripetal focus one of working with similars. He saw both as valid. To explain further, if you wanted to work in an expansive, outgoing, centrifugal way with yourself, your focus would be to heal with opposites, and work with sending energy from your core outward to your periphery, in all the ways we have described (see chapter 8). If you had a fever, you might use cold cloths (an opposite) to bring it down. You might also use bodywork on yourself that directs the energy outward. If you were to work with yourself in a receptive, inward returning centripetal way, you would focus on healing like with like, and work with the part of the cyclical process which moves from your outer edges back in to your core. Using a receptive centripetal approach with the same fever, you might choose to use an inflammatory homeopathic like belladonna, and move into the fever with the inward-oriented meditation given in chapter 4, or one from chapter 8. Both approaches, of course, can be successfully used in a course of healing. (10)

INTEGRATION:

As our "day" of self-healing together comes to a close, I'd like to invite you to consider creating your own self-care plan. Inevitably these change as we do, and yet in this moment you may be seeing and realizing things about your-self that could serve you for a while to come. Here is a chance to record your insights and musings. Fill out as much of this care plan as you feel ready to consider.

SELF-CARE PLAN

My name:_____

Today's date:

What I know works well for me:

MY PULSES: Right strong   Left strong

Balanced, both strong   Balanced, both weak

How might I respond to these, for effective healing?

ELEMENTS I would like to use more in my healing:

   earth   water   fire

   air   space

How I could do this:

SELF-CARE PLAN, p.2

CURRENTS: I feel most connected with:

East-West   Spiral   Long Lines

One way I could create a freer flow of energy through my currents would be:

If I were going to use MOVEMENT in healing, I'd like to play with:

On a scale of 1 (low) to 10 (high),

I'd rate my prana_____tejas_____ojas_____

If I wanted to change this, I could:

My time in MEDITATION is:

adequate   satisfying   too much

enough for me   zero   minimal

If I wanted to change this, I could:

SELF-CARE PLAN, p.3

Overall, my sense is: I need to cleanse.
                     I need to build.
                     I'm happy maintaining.

If I were going to shift my food choices I would:

Again, thinking about my pulses, the following seems
most true for me:

   I could let myself be more expansive.

   I could spend more time quietly receiving.

   I'm pretty balanced, in terms of my input and output.

In working with the step-down of energy, I see my life
purpose is to:

and I am here to create:

If I were my own healer, I would give myself this closing
acknowledgement with love and humor:

CHAPTER SYNOPSIS:
HEALING:
How much do you want to integrate?
How much are you willing to share?

RESOURCES IN HEALING

Stone, *Polarity Therapy*, vols. I & II (see footnotes).

Bhattacharyya, Benoytosh, *Gem Therapy*, revised and enlarged by A.K. Bhattacharya, Firma KLM Private Limited, Calcutta, 1981.

Chakravarti, Sree, *A Healer's Journey*, Rudra Press, Portland, OR, 1993, about mudras, also color: p. 203-219.

Lad, Vasant D., *The Complete Book of Ayurvedic Home Remedies*, Harmony Books, New York, 1998, about gems: p. 275-280.

X.

———•———

REST

TAMAS: Letting in Life, and Death. Completing.
Acknowledging our Wholeness.

*"Life is the expression of love in sound waves and energy
currents, throughout the creation and in man."*
STONE, HEALTH BUILDING, P. 15

It's time to close now. It is the end of our day together. I
thank you for joining me here and exploring together. And
I ask for the highest good for all sentient beings as all of us
journey off, singly and together, on our ways. May we open
to our deepest purpose and rest in that purpose.

Namaste!

APPENDIX:
MISCELLANEOUS NOTES TO PRACTITIONERS:

A "FAMILY-COUNSELING APPROACH" TO THE BODY AND MOVEMENT:

Both Polarity Therapy and Ayurveda can be adapted to use with other systems of healing, such as acupuncture, osteopathy, chiropractry, other forms of bodywork and movement, counseling, homeopathy, and Western medicine. How you apply the concepts of the energy currents or the doshas will depend on the sort of practice you have and your own affinity with these principles. Each practitioner develops their own perspective on the systems and how to apply it most effectively with themselves and others. For example, Rolfers or osteopaths are likely to be drawn to the structural applications of the work.

As a Polarity practitioner who has also trained in counseling, I have found myself gravitating toward what might be called, a "family-counseling" approach to Polarity Therapy. I like to explore how all the parts of the body relate to the whole. One can listen to each part of the body involved in an issue, trusting that it is important and needs to be heard. For those of you familiar with counseling language, the "designated patient" would be the part of the body that is offering a challenge, like the "presenting symptom" in medicine. And yet, as in family counseling, the presenting difficulty or designated patient is only part of the picture. There are brothers and sisters, mother and father, that is, other parts of the body involved in the current difficulty in some way. I'd like to explain more about this briefly.

I first began to notice these family-like relationships and how they could be used to support healing when a client came to me with a chronically frozen shoulder. The shoulder's mobility had been reduced to as little as 15% of its range of motion. When I checked in with the shoulder, by putting my hand on it and listening, it felt isolated and alone. I asked my client if this felt true to him, which it did.

We then proceeded to work together to bring the shoulder "back into the fold", so to speak, working with Polarity relationships between the shoulder and other parts of the body. Over the next two to three months of weekly sessions, my client regained roughly 75% of his range of motion in his shoulder. When we quit our work together, he was still slowly yet steadily improving.

MORE ABOUT PRANA, OJAS, AND BURNOUT:

This is a discussion for practitioners related to the material in chapter 3. Practitioners can also suffer imbalances in prana, tejas, and ojas. It is important to be able to identify imbalances in ourselves and our clients and deal with the situation appropriately. In the practitioner, a situation of high prana with low ojas can simply look like burnout. You may feel revved and initially exhilarated after giving a session, then find it hard to relax. Paradoxically, while you feel restless, you may also feel tired. (This tired wired feeling can also arise if you are short in the nutrient magnesium.)

In terms of clients, in a Polarity Therapy bodywork session, energy often builds up and releases in muscle twitches or spasms. This is normal. However, if prana or tejas are building up in your client to such a noticeable extent that it looks like a major episode of nervous discharge is imminent or in process, you have choices to make.

Polarity practitioners have different views on this discharge. Some consider it a healthy discharge of energy, which helps rebalance the system, which it can be. If you are working with trauma in the way Dr. Peter Levine does in his Somatic Experience work, twitching, violent shaking, changes in breathing can all signal the emergence of old trauma seeking to rebalance itself. If you are skilled in these methods, you may choose not to slow down the experience and instead support it. (see RESOURCES in chapter 3 and BIBLIOGRAPHY)

If you are not experienced in trauma work, however, there are a few simple things you can do, if the discharge becomes so strong it is upsetting to your client. People with a history of kundalini experiences, head injury, or depleted resources seem to be more prone to these more extreme experiences. The nervous system needs to be supported and the head needs to be kept cool. One can help one's client by having them get off the table, get their feet on the ground (literally) and make sure their head (fire oval) is cool. Literally, dunking one's head in cold water can help, or you can use a cooling rose water spray to the head. Immersing oneself completely in water, if possible, can also be helpful. However, simply getting the head under cool running water is often all that is needed. Usually you want the head to be cool and the feet to be warm. (This remedial approach is based on Ayurvedic and Tantric perspectives.)

Many of us may never encounter such an extreme reaction, and yet some of us will. My concern is that we invite this difficult possibility unless we adequately support ojas (see chapter 3). If we or our clients are run-down, rest is important. Discharge for the sake of drama is stupid, and can be hard on the nerves (literally!). For Polarity Therapy to be truly effective, we need to support ojas first. Resourcing techniques, such as those presented with SynergyDance in chapter 2, are an essential part of a healthy session, and support the development of ojas.

Sometimes prana and tejas can build up in relationship to a lot of spiritual practice, such as chanting or breath work. I have also seen prana and tejas build to high levels in some people when feelings accumulate, or when strong emotion is being experienced related to present conditions. In my experience to date, the charge that builds up in these situations does not seem to relate to old trauma, but simply is an imbalance in prana, tejas, and ojas. In these situations, the above methods can be helpful for re-establishing a healthy balance between the three energies. You will know that what you have suggested is working if your client calms down and feels better, more grounded, and not overly-stimulated.

Note: I am indebted here to the teaching of Dr. Robert Svoboda, Ayurvedic physician, in his workshop on rejuvenation given in Albuquerque, NM, spring, 1998. Any errors in understanding or application are, of course, my own.

APPENDIX: KEY DIFFERENCES BETWEEN AYURVEDIC AND POLARITY NUTRITION:

This section is included for people serious about pursuing more of a comparison of Ayurvedic and Polarity nutrition. Be forewarned: they do not always agree, and their contradictions can create bewilderment. If you are hard-core curious with questions, you may find this interesting. If you're already struggling to get clear about all that's been presented or you're just not that interested in nutrition, I'd recommend skipping this section. You can live without it.

While both Ayurveda and Polarity honor that each of us has a unique constitutional make-up, and both suggest eating according to our constitution, how to do this is significantly different between the two methods. Basically, Polarity's energetic nutrition balances thru similars, while Ayurvedic nutrition balances thru opposites.

To explain further on this point: if you are a fiery type, or Pitta in Ayurvedic terms, Ayurveda would suggest balancing your fire through the consumption of cooling tastes, namely sweet, bitter, and astringent foods. *You are a hot type, let's cool you down. (Ayurveda).* This balancing through opposites might include basmati rice or tapioca (sweet), or greens (bitter) or legumes (which have some astringency quality in them), as sweet, bitter, and astringent taste are all considered cooling in Ayurveda.

A Polarity Therapist would think about this in an entirely different way. She or he would look at your fiery nature and think, *this person needs more fiery foods, because they are fiery, it is their nature. (Polarity)* Beans and grains would still be recommended, but because they are considered "fiery" in this system. Because each person needs a balance of the elements, your Polarity therapist wouldn't object to you eating greens (watery) or tapioca (watery, dairy), they would simply want to make sure you got enough fiery foods. Very different, yes?

The two systems also have a different way of approaching oils. In Ayurvedic cooking, the first step in the preparation of many dishes is to heat up a small amount of oil in a skillet and warm spices in it, to activate the medicinal qualities of the herbs. Then the rest of the ingredients in the dish are added to this hot oil. The heated oils can help lubricate the digestive tract and calm excess gas, when used in moderation.

An excess of cooked oils will help neither the liver nor the GI tract as a whole, which was Stone's point. In an affluent nation where 40% of our calories come from fat, much of it heated, and most of it non-essential, Stone saw cooked oils as a burden to an already over-burdened liver. He avoided the use of heated fats, including those naturally occurring in nuts and dairy, in both his Purifying and Health Building regimes, only using it in the Gourmet Vegetarian protocol. One contradiction to this is his apparent recommendation of cheeses for health building. Any dairyman or old-fashioned cook knows that milk must be heated to make cheese.

But an excess of "raw" oils, as uncooked oils are called in Ayurveda, can also lead to problems, lowering digestive fire and slowing the motility of the villi. Villi are the cilia that line the small intestine, providing crucial absorptive sites in the uptake of nutrients from the digestive tract into the bloodstream. Ayurveda would generally look askance at a liver flush that includes 1/4 cup or more of oil in one sitting. The concern would be that doing this on a regular basis would slow digestion, rather than help cleanse it. An excess of fats also provides calories better gotten from protein-rich or complex carbohydrate foods. A little oil goes a long way, in each system.

On the other side of the coin, when I was in practice as a nutritionist, I saw individuals who had so faithfully adhered to a fat-free regime, that their bowels were having troubles moving. Here, adequate fluids and adequate fat, to lubricate the gut, are important. It could be as simple as a tablespoonful of cold-pressed olive or flax oil, or a little ghee.

To address another issue, both systems see a correspondence between the elements and taste. However, Polarity associates one element with each taste, while Ayurveda considers each taste a combination of two elements. Some of these correspondences agree with one another, others do not. These differences are included for your information in the following tables:

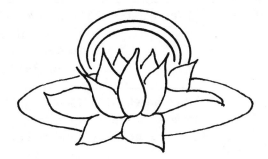

AYURVEDIC NUTRITION
SIX TASTES:

TASTE (elemental correspondence)	Example	Effect
SWEET (earth and water)	raisins, banana, sweeteners, well-chewed grains	Building. Adds moisture, coolness, and heaviness to the body.
SOUR (earth and fire)	lemon, citrus, umeboshi plum, vinegar, pickles, yogurt, buttermilk	Building. Adds moisture and warmth to the body.
SALTY (water and fire)	sea vegetables, sea food, salt, tamari	Building. Strengthens digestive fire. Warming, holds in water, can increase heaviness.
BITTER (air and ether)	leafy greens, some medicinal herbs	Cleansing. Strengthens the liver, cools the body, purifies the blood. Light and cool.
PUNGENT (fire and air)	chiles, garlic	Cleansing. Stimulates digestive fire, warmth. Hot, light action. Drying.
ASTRINGENT (air and earth)	witch hazel, unripe banana, persimmon	Cleansing. Contracting. Drying. Cold and light in action.

(reference: Ayurveda: Morningstar & Desai, *The Ayurvedic Cookbook*, p. 21-26)

ENERGETIC POLARITY NUTRITION:
FOUR TASTES:

TASTE (elemental correspondence)	Example	Effect
SWEET (earth)	fats, starches, sugars, honey	Earthy, adds weight. "Easily assimilated, slower in elimination"
SOUR (air)	acid fruits & juices, yeast, unprocessed cheeses, yogurt, buttermilk, acidophilus	Airy. Oxidizing. In excess, can increase fermentation & stiffness.
SALTY (water)	sea water, celery, cucumber, leafy vegetables, squash	Watery. Cleansing to the skin and mucus membranes, flushing accumulated sediments out.
BITTER (fire)	leafy greens, also foods with latent sprouting capacity, like: oats, peanuts, corn, sunflower seeds, & legumes	Fiery. Stimulates digestion, tonifying.

(reference: Polarity: Stone, *Polarity Therapy*, vol. I , bk. 3, p. 108-112.)

In looking at the elements as they manifest in food, in Ayurveda, the elements manifest as taste (see above) and also to some extent as state, that is, solid, liquid, temperature, gas. Stone in his development of Polarity energetic nutrition also looked at food and the elements in terms of state, a liquid food being watery, etc. And yet he didn't give ether any correspondence with taste. The ether element is considered in a number of ways in Polarity nutrition. For some therapists, it manifests as the space one creates in which to eat, and the way food is prepared and presented, i.e., "creating a good space". For others, such as nutritionist and Polarity Therapist James Champion, RPP, there are specific foods that embody ether, such as sprouts or quinoa. Champion has created a fascinating system of his own, based on Stone's original work, yet incorporating color and other components as well. This approach seems to work well for many. (See RESOURCES, chapter 5)

So how to choose between the Ayurvedic and Polarity systems for yourself? It depends on your needs. If you are looking for a simple, easy to follow vegetarian program and are basically fairly healthy, Polarity energetic nutrition plans are likely to serve you well. If you are attracted to complexity and enjoy juggling a number of factors in a healing diet, or you have a more serious illness, I would usually turn to Ayurveda for nutritional insight. Each approach has its strengths, and yet they are distinctly different. To use them together takes fortitude, patience, and a good dose of humor, in my view.

APPENDIX: DR. RANDOLPH STONE: A TIME LINE:

Feb. 26, 1890—Rudolf Bautsch (Randolph Stone) born in Engelsberg, Austria, the youngest of six children in a Catholic family.

1892—Rudolf's mother dies.

1903—emigrates to the US with his father and sister, arriving in Chicago on the 4th of July. They settle ultimately in Elgin, Illinois.

Early 1910s—studies to be a Lutheran minister at Concordia College in St. Paul, Minnesota. Travels and works as a machinist out West.

1914—receives degrees in osteopathy, chiropractry, naturopathy, naprapathy, and neuropathy from the State Board in Chicago. He is granted an O.P. (other practitioner's) license, the degree of the day for drugless healing methods.

1916—marries Mrs. Anna L. Stone, a Danish divorcee twenty years his senior, head nurse of the Lindhlar Nature Cure Sanitorium.

1919—at his wife's urging, changes his name to Randolph Stone.

1914—early 1970's—maintains an active practice in Chicago, where he is also a member of Manly P. Hall's Philosophical Research Society, the Masonic Lodge, and a respected student of Hindu, Rosicrucian, and Sufi teachings.

1935—Anna Stone dies.

1945—reads Dr. Julian Johnson's book The Path of the Masters which introduces him to the practice of Sant Mat. Later this year he is initiated into this path. He adopts a rigorous vegetarian diet as recommended for the practice. 1954-1957—publishes first works about Polarity Therapy, continues practice.

Early 1970's—closes practice in Chicago, and begins teaching multi-day seminars about his work across the U.S.

1973—retires completely to be with his teacher Charan Singh in India.

Dec. 9, 1981—dies in India.

Reference: *Polarity Therapy*, vol. II, p. 233-237

APPENDIX: PERSONAL SELF CARE RECIPES:
Based on the work of Melanie Sachs, *Ayurvedic Beauty Care*

Homemade lotions and potions let you know just what you are putting on and in your body. I got interested in making my own when I learned that propyl, phenyl, and methyl groups in common cosmetics like toothpaste and shampoo may hold toxic metals in the body, delaying their release and cleansing. People dealing with chemical sensitivity or metal poisoning especially can benefit from this "fast" from chemicals. Unfortunately, while natural grocery stores offer a wide-array of chemical-free foods, they often have body care aisles full of these additives.

Melanie Sachs has pioneered the use of Ayurvedic and Tibetan formulas in personal care. Her book, *Ayurvedic Beauty Care*, includes many more recipes.

A TOOTH POWDER:

1 c. sea salt
3 tsps. sandalwood (purifying, calms excess fire)
3 Tbsps. turmeric (tightens gums, purifies blood, antiseptic)
6 Tbsps. amla powder (very rich source of vit. C)
3 Tbsps. powdered neem leaves = one large handful (potent anti-microbial, calms excess fire)
Dash of black pepper (to stimulate the gums, also disinfectant)
Some calcium powder (optional, I use 6 capsules)

Melanie recommends applying the powder in a circular motion close to the gums over the gum line. Or you can rub it on sore spots with your fingers. The powder can also be used with your regular toothpaste, to add a healing effect.

Tongue scrapers: can be as simple as a teaspoon, or can be purchased through Banyan Trading Company, 1-800-953-6424 or Lotus Brands, 1-800-548-3824.

Oil: one good option is Spectrum brand unrefined organic sesame.

BASIC HERBAL CLEANSING POWDER:

12 Tbsps. chickpea flour (available in natural groceries as garbanzo flour, or in Indian groceries)
3 Tbsps. ashwagandha (available in bulk as Indian herb at natural groceries, etc.)
1 1/2 Tbsps. licorice root powder
Pinch of turmeric ("to brighten the skin", make you shine like the sun)*

To use this cleansing powder, put a little in your hand or a dish and moisten with warm water. Gently rub on to your face, washing it off with a washcloth or loofah. Follow with moisturizing cream.

*Melanie remarks on my version of this recipe that turmeric works best if you are dark-skinned (though I am pretty pale, myself). She observes that if you are white-skinned, you may risk "shining like an orange". For fair folks wishing to look other than fruit-like, she recommends a drop of tea tree oil instead, with the mixing water. It has the same antiseptic benefit.

NATURAL MOISTURIZING CREAM:

1 small stalk of aloe vera, peeled, or 1 Tbsp. aloe vera gel
1 1/2 oz. jojoba oil
1/2 oz. cocoa butter or shea butter
1 oz. rose water
Dash orange water
2 400 iu capsules of vitamin E, pierce, squeeze into blender
Up to 20 drops of pure essential oil, such as geranium oil and sandalwood oil, or whatever you like

Melt the cocoa butter in a small pan over low heat. Remove from heat and blend with the rest of the ingredients in a blender until creamy. Store in sealed glass container, in the refrigerator.

SIMPLE HAIR CONDITIONER:

Beat together in an unbreakable cup:

1 egg
Juice of half a lemon, or 1 Tbsp. apple cider vinegar (lemon smells better)
A few drops of essential oil for aroma (optional)

After washing your hair, massage the egg rinse into your hair and scalp and leave on for a few minutes before rinsing thoroughly with cool water. Adds protein, shine, friendly pH.

MEDICATED SALVE:

Medicated ghees or *ghritas* are a time-honored Ayurvedic remedy for rejuvenation. CAUTION: If you are going to use a ghrita like this internally, it would only be with the recommendation of an Ayurvedic physician, to be safe. It is important to be free of ama, waste. If you have a coated tongue, this would be one indicator of ama, and you would not use this internally.

This vegetarian herbal ghee was originally designed as a building formula. It is based on an original formula for asthi dhatu from Dr. Marc Halpern, president of the California College of Ayurveda. However, with modifications over the years, I've found it makes an excellent, if slightly odd, external salve, which strengthens most of the dhatus (tissues), including bone, nerve, and reproductive tissue. One to two teaspoons can be used externally safely in most situations; I would not use it in cases of fibroids, other growths, or tumors.

Medicated ghees like these can be fun to make, if you have a spare couple of hours to dawdle in your kitchen, and they are effective. One popular Ayurvedic ghrita is brahmi, made with gotu kola, to brighten the mind and memory. This particular recipe follows the standard formulation for ghritas, which is 16 parts water to 4 parts oil or ghee to 1 part herbs. Here we're using 8 cups total water, 2 cups total oil and ghee, and 1/2 cup herbs.

Simmer together for an hour in a heavy-bottomed stainless steel saucepan, or until the total fluid is reduced to 4 cups:

3 pieces organic kombu (seaweed) (optional, excellent source of minerals, including calcium)
8 c. water
2 Tbsps. gokshura (optional, good in kidney weakness) *
2 Tbsps. ashwaganda (especially strengthening to the male reproductive system)
1 Tbsp. shatavari (especially strengthening to the female reproductive system)
1 Tbsp. bala (supports the nerves)
1 Tbsp. galangal, chopped (optional, stimulates absorption and circulation of the herbs)
1 1/2 tsps. triphala
Scant tsp. cumin
Scant tsp. coriander

Strain out the herbs and seaweed and add:

1 c. organic ghee
1 c. extra virgin olive oil or sesame oil

if you are making a medicated salve for the bones.

If you are using this as a rejuvenative for the nerves or glands or as an externally applied aphrodisiac, use all ghee = 2 cups.

It's important to keep it going on a low heat. You can stir with a wooden spoon to keep it from sticking on the bottom. You are inviting the medicinal potencies of the herbs to enter the ghee in the presence of the water. When the ghrta is done, all the water is cooked off, just as it is when making ghee. This could take another hour. At this point you will have a thick medicated ghee that can be filtered through a dry stainless steel strainer into a glass or stainless steel jar. You should end up with close to two cups of ghrta, equivalent to the 2 cups of oil you began with. When cool, you can put it in a plastic squeeze container for easy abhyanga, to massage into those achy bones.

* This Ayurvedic herb has also been found to be an excellent source of natural testosterone, strengthening to both men and women. Research is being done on its role in alleviating chronic fatigue.

This ghee is appropriate for both sexes.

An excellent source for high-quality Ayurvedic herbs is Banyan Trading Company, 1-800-953-6424

ALMOND REJUVENATIVE MILK:

There are versions of this in both *Ayurvedic Cooking for Westerners* and *The Ayurvedic Cookbook*. Here is one way to build the tissues:

Soak overnight:

8 almonds in 1 cup pure water (save it)

In the morning, take a deep breath and peel all of them. Grind them finely in a blender or food processor or food mill, and then add:

the soaking water, plus
1/2 cup fresh milk, or rice or soy milk (optional, building)
dash of saffron (except in pregnancy)
dash of cardamom
pinch of Stevia or 1 tsp. of honey

Enjoy!

APPENDIX: MORE ABOUT ASTROLOGY AND MOVEMENT:

If you have a copy of your natal horoscope, you can begin to play with movement in a more focused way to heal tensions in both your psyche and body. Basically your astrological horoscope is a blueprint of the skies when you were born. Each of the planets, the signs, and their locations in the heavens at your birth time and place has a relationship to you in some way. One way to begin to get more familiar with your own chart and free up held-in energy at the same time, is to move with your horoscope.

First off, each planet evokes a particular energy. Traditionally Mars is considered assertive and energetic, Venus loving and graceful, Jupiter generous and expansive, to give a few resonances. Each planet is located in your natal chart in a particular sign. The combination of all the planets in these signs is unique to you. So for example, if you have Mars in Sagittarius, you might expect to discover some assertive energy in your thighs (See ASTROLOGY AND MOVEMENT chart for these associations). If you wanted to explore this, you could close your eyes, get in any position that felt comfortable to you, and begin to imagine you are expressing this energetic feeling through your thighs. A familiar song might come to you, or you might find yourself humming or moving in silence. Let yourself move as a way to become more familiar with this energy inside of you.

Perhaps you don't have Mars in this position, it's in Taurus, instead. You could do the same process, expressing assertive energy through your neck. (See ASTROLOGY AND MOVEMENT chart that follows for the associations). Or if your Mars is located in Gemini, it would be your shoulders that get to express this energy. You follow?

You can enact your full horoscope, in as much or little time as you want to take to play with it. Locate the position of each planet, then express the energy of that planet in the part of the body related to the sign in which it is located. You can start with the sun or moon and move through all the planets of our solar system. If you find this has meaning for you, and gives new insights, dance on! For example, you might want to explore the relationship of one planet to another, such as the Moon and Pluto. For example, if you had the Moon in Pisces and Pluto in Cancer, you could begin to move your feet in a way expressive of the fluidity and feelings of the Moon in Pisces. You could then let your heart and chest join in, moving from the deepest place you can contact (Pluto in Cancer). As you move these parts of your body, thoughts or feelings or sensations may arise. It is okay to notice them, and let them lead to healing.

ASTROLOGY AND MOVEMENT

PLANET	QUALITY OF ACTION OR MOVEMENT	NATURAL SIGN	BODY ZONE
Sun	essential, moving from your sense of self, your core	Leo	solar plexus
Moon	emotive, feeling, fluid	Cancer	breast, heart
Mercury	cerebral (moving from the mind or nervous system)	Gemini	shoulders
Venus	loving, graceful	Taurus (and) Libra	neck kidneys-adrenals
Mars	assertive, energetic	Aries	head
Jupiter	generous, expansive	Sagittarius	thighs
Chiron	focused, in the moment	Virgo	gut, bowels
Saturn	structured, contractive	Capricorn	knees
Uranus	spontaneous, inventive	Aquarius	ankles
Neptune	dreamy	Pisces	feet
Pluto	deep, profound, intense	Scorpio	pelvis, reproductive organs

(1)

For example, one client noticed as she moved her feet (Moon in Pisces) and her solar plexus (Pluto in Leo), that her personal feelings (Moon in Pisces) didn't feel as important as the deep connection with group consciousness that she felt in her solar plexus (Pluto in Leo). She could feel as she moved that she put more importance on the larger movements of our times, than she did her own feelings. This was neither good nor bad, just surprising to her. Her experience was that Pluto in Leo was located near her core, the solar plexus, while the Moon in Pisces was so far away, way down there in her feet. She hadn't realized this relationship inside her until she began to move it. Once she noticed it, she could see how she organized certain parts of her life in response to this unspoken reality. The choice of whether she wanted to continue to organize her life in this way now became a conscious one.

Polarity bodywork sessions can also be developed around these same relationships. For example, a T-square between Saturn, Pluto and Mars in your chart in the signs of Libra, Cancer and Capricorn could be worked on physically. Check out the energetic relationships between your kidneys (you can contact them with your hands on your back near your waist), heart and knees.

If you want to take this even further, you can do the movements that come to you in relationship to each planet, then look at the house in which this planet is located. If, for example, Pluto were located in your tenth house, the house of career and profession, your work would have to engage you deeply, or else you would be likely to feel frustrated and dissatisfied (see House chart that follows). Notice the kind of movements you make as you express the energy of Pluto. This may give you clues as to the ways you can work which will feel most satisfying professionally.

ASTROLOGICAL HOUSES AND THEIR MEANINGS

First	Personality, body, physical vitality
Second	Finances, resources (movable), values
Third	Our day-to-day mind, learning, communications, short journeys, siblings, neighbors, teaching
Fourth	Our home, intimate private self, family, tradition, real estate
Fifth	Play and amusement, creativity, self-expression, children, love affairs, gambling
Sixth	Service, day to day work, employees, health, nutrition, small animals
Seventh	Marriage, partnerships, one-to-one relationships, therapeutic relationships, known enemies, conflicts, lawsuits
Eighth	Death, sex, inheritance, other people's resources (and values)
Ninth	Our inspirational spiritual mind, philosophy, religion, spiritual practice, the law, long journeys
Tenth	Our career or profession, social status, honor, reputation, our parents, dealings with people who have authority over us
Eleventh	Our friends, important groups, our hopes, wishes, and ambitions
Twelfth	Our deep past, secrets, hidden relationships, our own undoing, sacrifice, karma, institution-alization or confinement, hidden limits

(1)

Astrologer and Registered Polarity Practitioner candidate Maureen O'Brien has observed that as the sun makes its way through the zodiac, it lights up each of our houses as it goes. This action naturally attracts our attention to this part of our lives, even if we are oblivious of astrology. So, for example, if you have Aquarius rising with Capricorn in the twelfth house, when the sun moves from Capricorn into Aquarius in late January each year, your focus may shift from darker twelfth house issues of your past, your hidden limits, and where you have been trapping yourself, to a lighter look at your personal needs in the present, your body and physical vitality (first house issues). Any transit can be explored through movement in the same way the natal horoscope can.

As you move with these patterns, long held emotions and ways of structuring your life may decide to release. You may even decide a new way of moving through your life is okay, even desirable.

It is not even necessary to have a horoscope to be able to apply these principles. For example, using triad work as described in chapter 2, you can begin to send support from the places that have resources to those in need of help. What do I mean? Let us use an imaginary example of a woman with constricted breathing or problems with her chest. Here is a place in need of support, the chest, a water zone. What are the other water zones in the body that might have resources to share? Looking at the table MOVE-MENT, THE BODY, AND THE ELEMENTS: TRIAD WORK in chapter 2, she sees the other two water zones are the pelvis and the feet. Knowing herself pretty well, she decides the feet are a safe place to start working. Putting one hand on her chest, the other hand would go to the feet. Or, if it was too hard to touch both places at once AND move, she could begin to simply move her chest and feet in ways that felt healing for her, sharing the energy of her feet with her heart. She might even begin to feel a therapeutic pulse, a rhythmic pulse, when she stops to notice how the two areas feel beneath her hands after her healing moves.

The skies manifest in our bodies, and we can move with their cycles for healing.

(1) References on tables: Morningstar, Werneke, and O'Brien, Traditional Western astrological associations, developed with Angela Werneke and Maureen O'Brien, Santa Fe, NM, 1999, see also Arroyo, *Astrology, Psychology, and the Four Elements*, p. 157-170, and 79-86.

See also:

Forrest, Stephen, *The Inner Sky*, the planets within us.

GLOSSARY OF POLARITY TERMS

air principle: see sattva.

anemia: a localized shortage of oxygen, due to lack of circulation to an area. Usually Stone was not referring to an overall low level of red blood cells as in a standard blood test when he mentioned this term.

bi-polar current: see long lines.

centrifugal current: any positively charged energy current flowing from the center outward (see *Polarity Therapy*, vol. II, p. 208), with its flow going from the brain to the extremities and back. An efferent energy associated with the outgoing breath and motor functions (movement), as well as daylight.

centrifugal stasis: deep congestion and swelling.

centrifugal treatment: working from the inside outward, from the core to the periphery.

centripetal current: any negatively charged energy current flowing from the surface inward. Associated with the in-breath and sensory awareness and the night. (See also *Polarity Therapy*, vol. I, book 2, p. 3)

centripetal spasm: surface tension or muscular contraction.

centripetal treatment: working from the ouside inward, from the periphery to the core.

core: the chakra system, including sushumna, ida and pingala.

depolarized: stagnant, without energy.

east-west current: see transverse current.

fire principle: see rajas.

five-pointed star: the geometric pattern formed by the neck, shoulders and hips, an expression of the yin water principle. See Stone, *Polarity Therapy*, vol. I, bk. 2, p. 16 and 17.

fresh food: raw food.

interlaced triangles: also known as the six-pointed star, it relates to the geometric pattern created in the body of the yang fire principle. The base of one anterior triangle begins at the hips and ends at the bridge of the nose, while the other base runs across the eyes and ends above the pubis. See Stone, *Polarity Therapy*, vol. I, bk. 2, p. 18 and Chitty and Muller, p. 137.

long lines: one of three primary energy currents, this one associated with the water principle. Dr. Stone considered them "direct currents from the five senses", (*Polarity Therapy*, vol. I, book 3, p. 29). Connected with up and down, top to bottom and return movements.

longitudinal currents: see long lines.

motor current: any current which pushes energy outward, usually located in the back (posterior) of the body. See Stone, *Health Building*, p. 137.

north pole: head, upper body, or anatomically a relatively superior area.

prana: life force carried by breath and food. Touch can also affect its circulation.

principles: the three principles of neutrality (air), expansion (fire) and contraction (water). Energy first manifests as the three principles before stepping down into the elements. See also gunas in the GLOSSARY OF AYURVEDIC TERMS.

rajas: out-going, expansive, the positive fire principle.

re-polarizing: to re-energize an area.

sattva: neutrality, the neutral blueprint of life, peace in balance, neutral air principle.

sensory current: any current which pulls energy in, usually located in the front (anterior) of the body. See Stone, *Health Building*, p. 137. Can also refer, with the motor currents, specifically to the long lines (see Stone, *Polarity Therapy*, vol. II, p. 102).

six-pointed star: more accurately called the interlaced triangles, see interlaced triangles.

south pole: feet, lower body, or an area which is anatomically relatively inferior.

spiral current: one of the three primary energy currents, an expression of the fire principle, radiating outward from the umbilicus, (navel) in a right-rotating spiral both front and back. Associated with forward and backward movement.

tamas: attractive, negative, yin, water principle.

transverse current: one of three primary energy currents, this one associated with the neutral air principle, moving down the chakras and out of the body, in two sideways moving spirals around the body, returning through the crown of the head. Connected with side to side motion.

triune energy: involving all three currents, principles, gunas.

umbilical current: see spiral current.

water principle: see tamas.

wireless anatomy: the energy network of the human body, including the currents.

GLOSSARY OF AYURVEDIC TERMS

abhyanga: oil massage, generously applied.

agni: digestive fire. Agni is also the sacred Hindu god of fire and the cosmic force of transformation.

ama: toxic wastes, usually created by low digestive fire and/or incomplete digestion, absorption, or elimination.

anandamaya kosha: the bliss sheath, part of the causal body.

annamaya kosha: the physical body, literally, the "food sheath".

artava: female reproductive tissue, one of the dhatus. Also used to denote one of the upadhatus of rasa, menstrual fluid.

asana: posture in yoga.

asthi: bone tissue, one of the dhatus.

ayurveda: the science of life and self-healing, also an art.

basti: medicated enema, either of oil or well-strained herbal tea; can be used for either cleansing or nourishment, depending on the ingredients and application.

bhakti: devotee, devotional.

bhasma: an Ayurvedic preparation which has been incinerated to ash, such as gems.

brahmi: gotu kola, an herb to strengthen the mind.

brihmana: building; nourishing, "making big, fat or strong".

dal: any split bean or pea, or any bean soup, in East Indian cooking.

danta: teeth, upadhatu of bone.

dasha: in Vedic astrology, a planetary period determined by our exact time of birth. Each of the planets watches over us for a specified number of years in a series of dashas throughout our lifetime. (pronounced with the emphasis on the second syllable)

dhatus: the seven essential tissues or "retainable structures" for health and life in Ayurveda.

dosha: one of three essential biological energies in Ayurveda: Vata, Pitta, and Kapha.

ghee: clarified butter, made by heating butter. An excellent carrier of nutrients and medicines to the deepest tissues, it stimulates flow and transformation, whereas butter stabilizes, congests. Important that it be organic.

ghrita or ghrta: medicated ghee, with herbs.

guna: attribute or quality. Often used to describe the mahagunas, qualities of mind, sattva, rajas, and tamas. Guna is also used to describe attributes such as rough, smooth, soft, and so forth.

ida: subtle channel arising from the left of the central channel, sushumna.

jyotish: Vedic astrology, the astrology of India.

kapha: earth-water dosha or constitution.

kardrara: muscle tendons, upadhatu of rakta, blood cells.

karma: effect or action.

kichadi: an Ayurvedic one-pot meal of mung beans, basmati rice, vegetables, and spices, often used for healing, in both cleansing and building.

langhana: cleansing; also fasting, drying up, reducing.

majja: nerve and bone marrow, one of the dhatus.

mala: one of the body's waste products, such as feces, urine, perspiration.

mamsa: muscle tissue, also includes the organs. One of the dhatus.

manomaya kosha: emotional sheath, part of the astral body.

mantra: healing sound, sacred sound which creates a specific energy.

marma: energy pressure point, used in Ayurvedic bodywork.

maya: an energy sheath around the body, enabling us to open to the divine. Also, illusion, the play of the universe.

meda: fat tissue, one of the essential dhatus.

mudra: sacred gesture, healing hand posture.

nadi: subtle energy channel.

nakshatras: the 27 or 28 constellations or dwelling places of the moon, used in ancient Indian astrology.

nasya: nasal cleansing with water, oil, and/or herbs.

neti: ceramic pot used in nasya, to rinse out nasal passages.

ojas: energy cushion, our vital life protector, immunity.

okasatmya: diets or lifestyles which have become non-harmful to the body through their regular, habitual use. Okasatmya describes how it is that one person can routinely eat something that would make another person quite ill.

pancha karma: the five cleansing practices of Ayurveda, vamana, virechana, basti, nasya, and rakta moksha.

pancha mahabhutas: the five great elements, ether, air, fire, water, and earth, which sustain all creation.

pingala: the subtle channel rising from the right of the central channel, sushumna.

pitta: fire-water dosha, the fiery dosha or constitution.

prakriti: constitutional type, determined at birth.

prana: subtle breath, life force, chi; the vital life force of the universe.

pranamaya kosha: the breath or vital sheath, part of the astral body close to the physical body.

pranayama: breathing practices, potent in balancing energy and health.

prasad: blessed food.

rajas: a quality of mind which evokes energy and action.

rajasic: a food or activity which promotes the fiery quality of mind. Fermented and spicy foods are both rajasic.

rakta: blood cell and lymph cell tissue, one of the dhatus.

rasa: plasma, the fluid portion of blood tissue, one of the dhatus. Also means feeling, fluid, sap, juicy life.

rasayana: a rejuvenative.

sadhana: spiritual practice.

sattva: a quality of mind which evokes clarity, harmony, and balance.

satmya: that to which we can become accustomed, which is healthy for us.

sattvic: a food or lifestyle or attitude which promotes clarity, non-harm, balance. Most freshly prepared vegetarian foods are sattvic.

shukra: male reproductive tissue, one of the dhatus.

sushumna: the central channel in the chakra network.

sira: blood vessel, upadhatu of blood cells.

smegma: everything from belly button lint to waste products of the genitals!

snaya: subcutaneous fat, upadhatu of meda, fat tissue.

srota: a vital channel in Ayurveda, a term which encompasses from the subtlest nadi to the largest passage of the GI tract.

stanya: colostrum, an upadhatu of rasa, plasma.

svedana: cleansing process of steaming, sweating.

tamas: a quality of mind intent on conservation and completion. Can be associated with darkness, inertia, and grounding.

tamasic: a food or lifestyle or practice which promotes tamas. Frozen food, microwaved food, and overeating can produce negative effects of tamas; whereas a freshly roasted onion made with love might simply help one ground.

tejas: our innate brilliance, luminescence, glow, creative fire.

tridosha: the three doshas of Vata, Pitta and Kapha as they work together.

tridoshic: substances or practices which simultaneously calm and support all three doshas.

triphala: literally, "three fruits". A strong tasting powdered herbal combination, quite useful for cleansing and tonifying the colon. By itself, can be a little astringent.

upadhatu: secondary tissue being built from the primary dhatu. Examples are colostrum, menstrual fluid, muscle tendons, head hair.

vaidya: Ayurvedic physician.

vata: air-ether dosha or constitution. Also, the five sub-doshas: *prana vayu:* vata that brings in prana from the environment through the nostrils, *udana vayu:* vata that moves energy up from the chest and torso out the mouth and nose, *samana vayu:* vata that nurtures digestive fire and circulation, *vyana vayu:* vata which supports circulation of the blood and lymph, and *apana vayu:* downward moving vata for elimination and birth. Ayurvedic physician Dr. Sunil Joshi gives a good description of all the sub-doshas in his informative book, *Ayurveda and Panchakarma* .

vijnanamaya kosha: applies to two energetics,1) the mental sheath, a part of the astral body related to thoughts and calculation, and 2) the intelligence sheath, a part of the causal body related to higher perceptions and will.

vikruti: the current imbalance of the doshas within the body, the current condition.

FOOTNOTES:

Note:

Dr. Stone's books were originally published separately. In 1985 CRCS Publications published an enlarged edition of *Health Building* that included *A Purifying Diet* and *Easy Stretching Postures*. *Polarity Therapy: The Complete Collected Works of Dr. Randolph Stone* was published by CRCS Publications in 1986 and 1987, including his more technical works. In this text, we have referred to the CRCS versions of Dr. Stone's works, by title, volume, book number, and page. If you have an older version of Dr. Stone's work, volume I, book 1 is *Energy*, volume I, book 2 is *The Wireless Anatomy of Man*, volume I, book 3 is *Polarity Therapy*. Volume II includes book 4, *The Mysterious Sacrum* and book 5 contains *Vitality Balance, Evolutionary Energy Charts, Polarity Therapy Principles & Practice, Energy Tracing, Private Notes for Polarity Therapy Students*, and *A Brief Explanation of the Emerald Tablet of Hermes*. Dr. Stone's books are readily available from CRCS Publications and the American Polarity Therapy Association.

About These Two Approaches:

1. Dr. Fred Smith, "A History of Ayurveda", talk, Southwest Yoga Conference, Austin, Texas, September 2, 1999.

2. Shubentsov and Gordon, *Cure Your Cravings*, p. 102-103.

3. Stone, *Polarity Therapy*, vol. II, p. 175.

4. Stone, *Polarity Therapy*, vol. I, bk. 1, p. 68.

5. Stone, *Polarity Therapy*, vol. I, bk. 1, p. 20).

6. Lad, *Ayurveda: The Science of Self-Healing*, p. 17.

7. Stone, *Polarity Therapy*, vol. I, bk,.1, p. 30, 32, 37. As a young Austrian immigrant to the United States, Stone learned his English primarily from the Bible, which definitely flavored his presentations throughout his professional life.

8. For a more detailed perspective on the step-down of energy from the gunas into matter as the elements, see Sills, *The Polarity Process*, p. 1–27, including charts on p. 9 and p. 23.

9. Stone, *Polarity Therapy*, vol. I, bk. 3, p. 51.

10. Stone, *Polarity Therapy*, vol. II, p. 208.

11. Stone, *Polarity Therapy*, vol. I, bk. 2, p. 2.

12. Stone, *Health Building*, p. 59.

13. Stone, *Polarity Therapy*, vol. I, bk. 3, p. 1-3.

14. Stone, *Polarity Therapy*, vol. II, p. 224.

15. Stone, *Health Building*, p. 76.

16. Stone, *Polarity Therapy*, vol. I, bk. 1, p. 42.

17. Stone, *Polarity Therapy*, vol. I, bk. 1, p. 40.

18. Observations of Cindy Rawlinson and James Said contributed greatly to my understanding of Dr. Stone and his work in this entire chapter, in conversations, January, 2000.

Chapter 1: WAKING

1. Stone, *Health-Building,* p. 142.

2. Stone, *Health Building,* p. 142.

3. Lopan Phurba Dorje, preliminary teachings on Tibetan Buddhism, assistant to Gyangteng Tulku Rinpoche, Santa Fe, Winter, 1999.

4. *Health Building,* p. 113.

5. Quote from Sills, *The Polarity Process,* p. 29. See also: Stone, *Polarity Therapy,* vol. I, book 2, p. 8 & Sills, *The Polarity Process,* p. 26-42.

6. Stone, *Polarity Therapy,* vol. I, book 2, p. 9.

7. Lad, *Ayurveda: The Science of Self-Healing,* p. 26-31.

8. Stone, *Polarity Therapy,* vol. I, bk.2, p. 84; *Health Building,* p. 121 and 106.

9. Stone, *Polarity Therapy,* vol. I, bk. 1, p. 53.

10. See particularly Svoboda, *Prakriti: Your Ayurvedic Constitution,* the whole book, as well as Morningstar and Desai, *The Ayurvedic Cookbook,* p. 8-20.

10. Stone, *Health Building,* p. 91.

Chapter 2: MOVEMENT

1. Stone, *Health Building*, p. 97.

2. Lee, Charmaine, in conversation, January 25, 2000.

3. Stone, *Polarity Therapy*, vol. I, bk. 3, p. 14.

4. Stone, *Health Building*, p. 11.

5. Stone, *Polarity Therapy*, vol. I, bk. 2, p. 65-66.

6. Stone, *Polarity Therapy*, vol. I, bk. 3, p. 11.

7. Stone, *Health Building*, p. 55.

8. Said, James, in conversations, January, 2000. Fazio, Damon in trainings, Sept. 1996, Albuquerque, NM.

9. Lee, Charmaine, Synergy Dance workshop, Albuquerque, NM, 1997, and Chitty & Muller, *Energy Exercises*, p. 14. More accurately, James Said has observed that the transverse current reveals itself in torsional and compressive-extension movements.

10. Said, James, ibid.

11. Lee, Charmaine, 1997 and Chitty & Muller, ibid. James Said associates the spiral current with side-to-side movements.

12. Lee, Charmaine, in conversation, January, 2000. In relationship to the movement of the long lines out of the chakras, James Said has said that they flow upward and downward from "in front on the right and in back on the left, according to the right hand rule".

13. Said, James, ibid.

14. Sills, *The Polarity Process*, p. 31.

15. Lee, 1997, and Chitty & Muller, *Energy Exercises*, ibid. James Said adds that their movements also relate to forward and backward direction.

16. Said, James has observed the strong way in which the currents create our place in three dimensional reality. However, he would say that the transverse current reveals itself in superior-inferior and torsional motion anatomically; the spiral current in side bending; and the long lines in forward and backward motion, as well as upward and downward moves.

17. Said, Jim and Cindy Rawlinson, conversations, January, 2000.

18. Feedback from Charmaine Lee was essential in developing an accurate approach to this current, January 2000.

19. Anderson, *Stretching*, p. 15. Also, for people working from a chair, Chitty & Muller have created a full routine of Polarity stretches, "Exercises in a Chair" in Energy Exercises, p. 135.

20. Stone, *Polarity Therapy*, vol. I, bk. 2, p. 84.

21. Stone, *Polarity Therapy*, vol. II, bk.5, p. 438.

22. Stone, *Polarity Therapy*, vol. I, bk. 1, p. 49, as well as conversation with Charmaine Lee, January, 2000.

23. Viniyoga, a profoundly healing system of yoga from India, would look at the preceding two postures in a little bit different way. Inhaling into a backbend would be considered building, *brihmana*, while moving into the fetal position with an exhale would be used for cleansing, *langhana*. Viniyoga was originated by the yogi Krishnamacharya in the early part of the twentieth century and is taught today by his son T.K.V. Desikachar, as well as talented teachers in the West. In Madras, sick individuals have the option of treating their illness with yoga at the Krishnamacharya Yoga Mandiram clinic, as an alternative or support to other medical approaches. For more information about this approach, see Desikachar, *The Heart of Yoga*; Kraftsow, *Yoga for Wellness*; and Rawlinson, *Yoga for the West*.

24. Stone, *Health Building*, p. 173, then p. 139.

25. Stone, *Polarity Therapy*, vol. I, bk. 1, p. 48-9 & *Health Building*, p. 175.

26. For many more skillfully directed therapeutic yoga moves, see Kraftsow, *Yoga for Wellness*.

27. Stone, *Polarity Therapy*, vol. I, bk. 2, p. 61.

28. There are a wide range of relationships possible in any of the moves. For much more information about this, see Chitty & Muller, *Energy Exercises*.

29. Stone, *Health Building*, p. 170.

30. Stone, *Health Building*, p. 182.

31. Stone, *Health Building*, p. 183.

32. Stone, *Polarity Therapy*, vol. II, p. 126.

33. Stone, *Health Building*, p. 180.

34. Chitty & Muller, *Energy Exercises*, p. 44-45.

35. Stone, *Health Building*, p. 158.

36. Stone, *Health Building*, p. 160-161.

37. Chitty & Muller, *Energy Exercises*, p. 31-32.

38. Stone, *Health Building*, p. 159.

39. Stone, *Health Building*, p. 171 & 181. If your shoulders feel like this is more than they can handle, the Owl in Chitty & Muller's *Energy Exercises*, p. 26-27 is a good warm-up to it, or a gentle alternative.

40. Stone, *Health Building*, p. 150-151 and 111-112.

41. Stone, *Health Building*, P. 108.

42. Lee, conversation about moving growth energy blocks with the currents, Jan. 25, 2000.

43. Charmaine Lee, Albuquerque, lecture and demonstration, May 1997; and at APTA national conference, workshop, Ellensville, New York, June 1999.

44. Laurie Forbes demonstrates the Polarity Therapy fire line in the fire moves shown here, in an original developmental movement, February 2000.

45. Stone, *Polarity Therapy*, vol. II, p. 52.

46. Stone, *Polarity Therapy*, vol. I, bk. 3, p. 24, 29, 37-42 for a start.

47. Stone, *Polarity Therapy*, vol. II, bk. 5, p. 7.

48. Chitty and Muller, *Energy Exercises*, p. 111.

49. Stone, *Polarity Therapy*, vol. II, p. 195. Stone also spoke frequently of the connection between freeing up the shoulders and its positive effect on the heart and nervous system, through the brachial plexus nerve. There is a good article about this by Mary Jo Ruggieri, PhD, RPP, "The Power of the

Brachial Plexus" in *Energy: The Newsletter of the American Polarity Therapy Association*, vol. XV, no.1, winter 2000.

Chapter 3: BREATH

1. Stone, *Polarity Therapy*, vol. I, bk 1, p. 61.

2. Pert, *Molecules of Emotion*, p. 186-7.

3. Stone, *Polarity Therapy*, vol. II, p. 132.

4. Charmaine Lee, in conversation, Jan. 25, 2000.

5. Stone, *Polarity Therapy*, vol. I, bk. 1, p. 2 and 3. (These effects, that Dr. Stone described fifty years ago, can now be readily seen through the physical technology of dark field microscopy.)

6. Stone, *Polarity Therapy*, vol. I, bk. 1, p. 57.

7. Stone, *Health Building*, p. 29.

8. Desikachar, *The Heart of Yoga: Developing a Personal Practice*, p. 138.

9. *Charaka Samhita*, vol. I, p. 386.

10. For more about calming Vata, see also Morningstar, *The Ayurvedic Cookbook*, p. 13-14.

11. For example, the Tibetan Buddhist practice of the Three Lights, a visualization/meditation process given in the sixteenth Karmapa's lineage as well as other Buddhist lines, specifically supports prana, tejas and ojas, as I understand them. It is also said in some schools of Tibetan Buddhism that there is a subtle prana, and that if one can strengthen the subtle prana, the physical prana will be benefited.

Again, if you are familiar with Tibetan Buddhism, you may be able to see a correspondence between prana, tejas and ojas, and the three kayas. Prana can be seen as a manifestation of dharmakaya, awareness-emptiness, and tejas as a manifestation of sambhogakaya, inner luminescence. Ojas may then correspond with nirmanakaya. While these are subtle energies, they also relate quite practically to our health and happiness.

12. Stone, *Polarity Therapy*, vol. I, bk. 2, p. 9.

13. "Physicist's back injury inspires scientific study of acupuncture", Debra Gordon, in *Albuquerque Journal,* December 28, 1998, C:1. Dr. Cho's studies have been published in the spring, 1998 issue of the Proceedings of the National Academy of Science.

14. There's a thoughtful article about Gandhi and his philosophy of "Renounce and enjoy," as it relates to our ozone-depleted world, "Joys R Us", Bill McKibben, originally printed in *Mother Jones,* Nov./Dec. 1999, reprinted in *Utne Reader,* Mar./April 2000. Or for a more hard-hitting, economic approach, see T*he Case Against the Global Economy,* Mander et al., eds.

15. "Heart, the seat of ojas", quote from *Charaka Samhita,* vol. I, p. 593. About the role of subtle prana in the heart, Gyangteng Tulku Rinpoche, teachings in Pagosa Springs, CO, and Santa Fe, NM, spring 1999.

Chapter 4: STILLNESS

1. Stone, *Health Building*, p. 26.

2. Stone, *Polarity Therapy,* vol. I, bk. 1, p. 47.

3. Stone, *Polarity Therapy,* vol. I, bk. 3, p. 5.

4. Stone, *Polarity Therapy,* vol. I, bk. 3, p. 26.

Chapter 5: NOURISHMENT

1. Murrieta Foundation, *Murrieta Hot Springs Vegetarian Cookbook,* p. 5-15.

2. Stone, *Health Building,* p. 76 & 91.

3. *Charaka Samhita,* p. 552-556 presents the healing benefits of meat. In another section of Charaka, the advantages of a non-violent lifestyle are given, namely, longevity.

4. Morningstar, *Ayurvedic Cooking for Westerners,* p. 10-15.

5. Sills, T*he Polarity Process,* p. 184 (from James Said), p. 159.

6. Stone, *Polarity Therapy*, vol. I, bk. 3, p. 110.

7. Stone, *Polarity Therapy*, vol. I , bk. 3, p. 111.

8. Stone, *Polarity Therapy*, vol. I, bk. 3, p. 108-116, vol. II, p. 202-203; Sills, *The Polarity Process*, p. 184.

9. Lad, Ayurveda: *The Science of Self-Healing*, p. 48-51.

Chapter 6: CLEANSING

1. *Charaka Samhita*, vol. IV, p. 161.

2. Joshi, *Ayurveda and Panchakarma*, p. 165-166.

3. *Charaka Samhita*, vol. II, p. 430, commentary.

4. *Charaka Samhita*, vol. II, p. 112.

5. For sample recipes, see Morningstar and Desai, *The Ayurvedic Cookbook*, which has a wide-range of therapeutic kichadis, p. 115-125, or Morningstar, *Ayurvedic Cooking for Westerners*, p. 121 for a basic kichadi.

6. Sharan, *Herbs of Grace*, p. 91.

7. Pitchford, *Healing with Whole Foods*, revised edition, p. 240.

8. Murrieta Foundation, *Murrieta Hot Springs Vegetarian Cookbook*, p. 21.

9. Stone, *Health Building*, p. 47.

10. Ibid.

11. Stone, *Health Building*, p. 88.

12. Stone, *Health Building*, p. 87.

13. Stone, *Polarity Therapy*, vol. I, bk. 2, p. 16-17.

14. Stone, *Polarity Therapy*, vol. I, bk. 2, p. 18.

15. Nadkarni, *Indian Materia Medica*, vol. I, p. 277.

16. Jensen, Derrick, "An Epidemic of Deception: Why We Can't Trust the Cancer Establishment, An Interview with Samuel Epstein", in *The Sun*, issue 291, March 2000.

17. Ward et al, 1989, cited in *Toxicological Profile for Aluminum*, U.S. Department of Health and Human Services, Public Health

Service, Agency for Toxic Substances and Disease Registry, TP-91/01, with thanks to Ronald E. Voorhees, MD, MPH, N.M. deputy state epidemiologist, spring, 1993.

18. Galland, *The Four Pillars of Healing*, p. 98-99, goes into detail on this. It is important to note that, to date, the research linking Klebsiella and joint pain has been associated primarily with ankalosing spondilitis, centered around the spine.

Chapter 6: CLEANSING HOME REMEDIES TABLES

1. All fresh vegetable juice recommendations are from Stone, *Health Building*, p. 73-75 unless otherwise noted.

2. Stone, *Health Building*, p. 52.

3. Stone, *Polarity Therapy*, vol. II, p. 209, for one example of this approach see vol. II, p. 126, figure 1.

4. Stone, *Health Building*, p. 52.

5. Stone, *Polarity Therapy*, vol. II, p. 210-211.

6. Stone, *Health Building*, p. 80.

7. Stone, *Health Building*, p. 74.

8. Stone, *Health Building*, p. 93, see also *Polarity Therapy*, vol. I, bk. 1, p. 59 and vol. II, p. 214.

9. Stone, *Health Building*, p. 69.

10. Stone, *Health Building*, p. 50, see also *Polarity Therapy*, vol. I, bk. 3, p. 91.

11. Stone, *Health Building*, p. 39.

12. Stone, *Health Building*, p. 82.

13. Stone, *Polarity Therapy*, vol. I, bk. 1, p. 72-3.

14. Stone, *Polarity Therapy*, vol. I, bk. 1, p. 83 and bk. 2, p. 38.

15. Stone, *Health Building*, p. 70.

16. Stone, *Polarity Therapy*, vol. I, bk. 2, p. 83.

17. Stone, *Polarity Therapy*, vol. I, bk. 3, p. 110, and *Health Building*, p. 45.

18. Stone, *Health Building*, p. 69.

19. Stone, *Health Building*, p. 48.

20. Stone, *Health Building*, p. 71.

21. Stone, *Health Building*, p. 121, how to: p. 134, see also *Wood Chopper*, p. 158.

22. Stone, *Health Building*, p. 70.

23. Stone, *Health Building*, p. 47.

24. Stone, *Health Building*, p. 90.

25. Stone, *Health Building*, p. 70.

26. Stone, *Health Building*, p. 87-88.

27. Stone, *Health Building*, p. 78 and 106.

28. Stone, *Health Building*, p. 42.

29. Stone, *Polarity Therapy*, vol. II, p. 57 for a specific exercise to relax the neck & shoulders.

30. Stone, *Health Building*, p. 88.

31. Stone, *Health Building*, p. 46.

32. Stone, *Health Building*, p. 44-45; for specific contacts to clear blocks in digestion and liver function, more easily done by another person, see *Polarity Therapy*, vol. I, bk. 2, p. 78.

33. Stone, *Polarity Therapy*, vol. II, bk. 5, p. 22.

34. Stone, *Health Building*, p. 42-43; countryside technique for relieving a headache, another person is needed to perform these simple moves: *Polarity Therapy*, vol. I, bk. 2, p. 58, chart # 49.

35. Stone, *Polarity Therapy*, vol. II, bk. 5, p. 86.

36. Stone, *Polarity Therapy*, vol. I, bk. 1, p. 81 & 83; bk. 2, p. 33; vol. II, p. 154 & 197.

37. Stone, *Health Building*, p. 178.

38. Stone, *Health Building*, p. 71.

39. Stone, *Health Building*, p. 70.

40. Stone, *Polarity Therapy*, vol. II, p. 214.

41. Stone, *Health Building*, p. 67-68.

42. Stone, *Health Building*, p. 179-180.

43. Stone, *Health Building*, p. 80.

44. Stone, *Health Building*, p. 68.

45. Stone, *Health Building*, p. 155 and *Polarity Therapy*, vol. I, bk. 2, p. 61 & 85. Stone wrote often about the relationship between the pelvis and the sinuses; correcting imbalances in the pelvis, revealed in part by a short leg, often helped a great deal.

46. Stone, *Health Building*, p. 68.

47. Stone, *Health Building*, p. 70.

48. Stone, *Health Building*, p. 68.

49. Stone, *Polarity Therapy*, vol. II, p. 167.

50. Stone, *Health Building*, p. 68.

51. Stone, *Health Building*, p. 51-52.

52. Stone, *Health Building*, p. 69.

53. Stone, *Health Building*, p. 70.

54. Stone, *Health Building*, p. 69.

55. Stone, *Health Building*, p. 68.

56. Stone, *Health Building*, p. 33-34.

57. Stone, *Health Building*, p. 69.

58. Stone, *Polarity Therapy*, vol. II, bk. 5, p. 102.

59. Stone, *Polarity Therapy*, vol. II, p. 191.

60. Stone, *Health Building*, p. 69.

61. Stone, *Health Building*, p. 49; *Polarity Therapy*, vol. I, bk. 2, p. 84.

62. *Health Building*, ibid.

63. Stone, *Health Building*, p. 121-122.

64. Stone, *Polarity Therapy*, vol. I, bk. 2, p. 24: chart #17.

65. Stone, *Polarity Therapy*, vol. I. bk. 3, p. 41, see also bk. 2, p. 30 & 31.

Chapter 7: BUILDING

1. Stone, *Health Building*, p. 126.

2. *Charaka Samhita*, vol. I, p. 374-378.

3. *Charaka Samhita*, vol. I, p. 381.

4. *Charaka Samhita*, vol. IV, p. 189.

5. Commentary in *Charaka Samhita*, vol. II, p. 430.

6. For more information about the three Polarity food processes, see Stone's *Health Building* and *Murrieta Hot Springs Vegetarian Cookbook*.

7. Discussion with Polarity teachers, former students of Dr. Stone, during teachers' forum, APTA national conference, Keystone, Colo., 1998.

8. *Charaka Samhita*, vol. I, p. 400.

9. Interview with Dr. Robert Svoboda, Ayurvedic physician, spring, 1998, Albuquerque, NM.

10. *Charaka Samhita*, vol. I, p. 181.

11. *Charaka Samhita*, vol. IV, p. 7-9.

12. *Earth Island Journal*, Winter, 1999-2000, p. 3.

13. Stone, *Polarity Therapy*, vol. I, bk 3, p. 111-112.

14. Erasmus, *Fats That Heal, Fats That Kill*, p. 48.

15. Morningstar, personal note as a practitioner: I have also seen the overall vitality and subsequent "charge" of a person suffer when they were short in vitamin B-12. One client's energy and ability to perceive energy noticeably improved after she took a series of vitamin B-12 shots for an underlying deficiency.

16. Interview, Robert Svoboda, ibid.

17. Interview, Robert Svoboda, ibid.

18. I want to express my appreciation here for Ayurvedic educators who have supported my understanding of Ayurvedic nutrition, through their teaching and work. These include: Dr. Virender Sodhi, Drs. Avinash and Bharati Lele, Swami Sada Shiva Tirtha, Dr. David Frawley, Dr. Vasant and Usha Lad, Drs. Sunil and Shalmali Joshi, Dr. Abbas Qutab, Patricia Hansen, Bri. Maya Tiwari, Dr. John Douillard, and Dr. Marc Halpern.

Chapter 7: BUILDING HOME REMEDIES TABLES

1. All fresh vegetable juice recommendations are from Stone, *Health Building*, p. 73-75 unless otherwise noted.

2. Stone, *Health Building*, p. 74.

3. Stone, *Health Building*, p. 144-146, for more information.

4. Stone, *Health Building*, p. 69.

5. Stone, *Health Building*, p. 82, and *Polarity Therapy*, vol. I, bk. 3, p. 108.

6. Stone, *Health Building*, p. 50 and 178.

7. Stone, *Health Building*, p. 74.

8. Stone, *Polarity Therapy*, vol. II, p. 53-56.

9. ibid.

10. Stone, *Polarity Therapy*, vol. II, p. 45, see also vol. I, bk. 3, p. 40-41.

11. ibid, p. 165.

12. ibid, p. 193.

13. ibid, p. 149.

14. ibid, p. 126.

15. Stone, *Health Building*, p. 49.

16. Stone, *Polarity Therapy*, vol. I, bk. 2, p. 44, 84-85; see also an excellent stretch, *Polarity Therapy*, vol. II, p. 182.

17. Stone, *Polarity Therapy*, vol. II, p. 148.

18. Stone, *Health Building*, p. 140.

19. ibid, p. 74.

Chapter 8: CREATIVE ACTION

1. Morrnah Simeona, founder, the Foundation of I, Self Identity through Ho'oponopono, classes in Santa Fe, NM, 1985-1988.

2. Stone, *Polarity Therapy*, vol. II, p. 209-213.

3. Stone, *Polarity Therapy*, vol. I, bk. 3, p. 116.

4. Kraftsow, *Yoga in Wellness*, p. 296-300.

5. See also Stone's comments, *Polarity Therapy*, vol. I. bk. 3, p. 35-36.

6. In Tibetan meditation practice, this mind-body relationship can be looked at not as a dichotomy with two participants, but rather as a trio, the three gates, usually translated body, speech and mind. I began to think of this in a different way when Dzog Chen teacher Namkai Norbu spoke on this topic recently in Santa Fe, August 27, 1999. He talked about the three gates to awareness being body, energy, and mind.

7. Stone, *Polarity Therapy*, vol. I, bk. 3, p. 12.

8. *Mind in Buddhist Psychology*, eds. Guenther & Kawamura. In some Tibetan Buddhist medicine texts, this view is not held. Often a feeling like anger or fear will be considered imbalancing and unhealthful, e.g., Ian Baker, *The Tibetan Art of Healing*.

9. Namkai Norbu, talk on Dzog Chen, Santa Fe, New Mexico, August 27, 1999.

10. Morningstar, educational process developed in 1987.

11. Stone, *Polarity Therapy*, vol. II, bk. 4, p. 42-44.

12. Stone, *Health Building*, p. 106.

13. Stone, *Polarity Therapy*, vol. I. Bk. 1, p. 49 and vol. II, bk. 4, p. 42.

14. Stone, *Polarity Therapy*, vol. II, bk. 4, p.42

15. General note about Vedic astrology: for those interested yet not trained in this art, studying the *dashas* is often a relatively quick and fruitful way to get valuable perspectives on the individual, her or his current focus, and ways of healing.

Chapter 9: HEALING: SUBTLE DIMENSIONS

1. Stone, *Polarity Therapy*, vol. I, bk. 3, p. 29 and bk. 2, p. 12.

2. Conversations, James Said, DC, RPP and Cindy Rawlinson, LAc, RPP, Jan. 13, 2000.

3. Stone, *Polarity Therapy*, vol. I, bk. 2, p. 14 and vol. II, p. 180-181.

4. The author's experience, as well as the experience of Shubentsov reported in *Cure Your Cravings.*

5. Stone, *Polarity Therapy,* vol. II, p.168.

6. Stone, *Polarity Therapy,* vol. II, p.174.

7. Stone, *Polarity Therapy,* vol. II, p.171.

8. Stone, *Polarity Therapy,* vol. II, p.170-175. Thanks also to Edith Hathaway, Vedic astrologer, for her cogent perspectives on this section. *Lal Kitab* is a book published in India with further information on this subject for those seriously interested.

9. Stone, *Polarity Therapy,* vol. I, bk. 3, p. 1-2, 31.

10. Ibid, plus conversations with Said and Rawlinson, Jan. 13, 2000.

BIBLIOGRAPHY:

Agnivesa, *C(h)araka Samhita,* Chowkhamba Sanskrit Series Office and Chaukhambha Orientalia, Varanasi, India, vols. I–IV, 1976 to 1993

Alon, Ruthy, *Mindful Spontaneity: Lessons in the Feldenkrais Method,* North Atlantic Books, Berkeley, CA, 1996

Anderson, Bob, *Stretching,* Shelter Publications, Inc., Bolinas, CA, 1980

Arewa, Caroline Shola, *Opening to Spirit: Contacting the Healing Power of the Chakras and Honouring African Spirituality,* Thorsons, London, 1998

Arroyo, Stephen, *Astrology, Psychology, and the Four Elements: An Energy Approach to Astrology and Its Use in the Counseling Arts,* CRCS Publications, Reno, NV, 1975

Ballentine, Rudolph, *Diet & Nutrition: a holistic approach,* The Himalayan International Institute, Honesdale, PA, 1978

Beaulieu, John, *Polarity Therapy Workbook,* BioSonic Enterprises, Ltd., New York, 1994

Bhattacharyya, Benoytosh, *Gem Therapy,* revised and enlarged by A.K. Bhattacharya, Firma KLM Private Limited, Calcutta, 1981

Blum, Jeanne Elizabeth, *Woman Heal Thyself: An Ancient Healing System for Contemporary Women,* Charles E. Tuttle Company, Boston, MA, 1995

Bodary, John R., compiler of *Index to the Polarity Writings of Dr. Randolph Stone,* the Polarity Center, 5824 Chase Road, Dearborn, Michigan, 48126, 1992

Buist, Robert, *Food Chemical Sensitivity,* Harper & Row, Sydney, Australia, 1986

Burger, Bruce, *Esoteric Anatomy: The Body as Consciousness,* North Atlantic Books, Berkeley, California, 1998

Calais-Germain, Blandine, *Anatomy of Movement,* Eastland Press, Seattle, WA, 1993, English edition

Cartwright, Lee, *SCtD (TM) Meditations: Transformational Tools for the Health Practitioner: An Introduction in Outline Form,* 1472 St. Francis Dr., Santa Fe, NM 87505

Chakravarti, Sree, *A Healer's Journey,* Rudra Press, Portland, OR, 1993

Chitty, Anna, *Energy Exercises* video, Polarity Press, 1721 Redwood Ave., Boulder, CO 80304, (303) 443-9847

Chitty, John and Anna, *Relationships and the Human Energy Field: Training Course Manual,* Polarity Center of Colorado, Boulder, CO, 1991

Chitty, John and Mary Louise Muller, *Energy Exercises: Easy Exercises for Health & Vitality* book, Polarity Press, 1721 Redwood Ave., Boulder, CO 80304, (303) 443-9847, 1990

Chopra, Deepak, *Perfect Health,* Harmony Books, New York, 1991

Colbin, Annemarie, *Food and Healing,* Ballantine Books, New York, 1986

Colbin, Annemarie, *The Book of Whole Meals,* Ballantine Books, New York, 1979

D'Adamo, Peter, *Eat Right for Your Type,* GP Putnam's Sons, New York, 1996

Davies, Stephen, and Alan Stewart, *Nutritional Medicine: The drug-free guide to better family health,* Pan Books, London, 1987

Dennison, Paul E. and Gail E., *Brain Gym: Simple Activities for Whole Brain Learning*, Edu-Kinesthetics, Inc., PO Box 3396, Ventura, CA 93006-3396

Desikachar, T.K.V., *The Heart of Yoga: Developing a Personal Practice*, Inner Traditions International, Rochester, VT, 1995

Erasmus, Udo, *Fats That Heal, Fats That Kill*, Alive Books, Burnaby, BC, Canada, 1993

Farhi, Donna, *The Breathing Book: Good Health and Vitality Through Essential Breath Work*, Henry Holt, New York, 1996

Flaws, Bob, *The Book of Jook: Chinese Medicinal Porridges, A Healthy Alternative to the Typical Western Breakfast*, Blue Poppy Press, Boulder, CO, 1998

Forrest, Stephen, *The Inner Sky*, ACS Publishers, 1989

Francis, John, *Polarity Yoga: A Series of Self-Help Exercises*, 1985, available through APTA, Boulder, CO

Frawley, David, *Ayurvedic Healing: A Comprehensive Guide*, Passage Press, Salt Lake City, Utah, 1989

Frawley, David, *Ayurvedic Healing Correspondence Course for Health Care Professionals*, Santa Fe, 1996, American Institute of Vedic Studies, PO Box 8357, Santa Fe, NM, 87504-8357

Frawley, David, *Yoga & Ayurveda: Self-Healing and Self-Realization*, Lotus Press, Twin Lakes, WI, 1999

Gagnon, Daniel and Amadea Morningstar, *Breathe Free: Nutritional and Herbal Care For Your Respiratory System*, Lotus Press, Twin Lakes, WI, 1991

Galland, Leo, *The Four Pillars of Healing: How the New Integrated Medicine—the Best of Conventional and Alternative Approaches—Can Cure You*, Random House, New York, 1997

Gordon, Richard, *Your Healing Hands—The Polarity Experience*, Unity Press, Santa Cruz, CA, 1978

Guenther, ed., *Mind in Buddhist Psychology*, a translation of Ye-shes rgyal-mtshan's "The Necklace of Clear Understanding" by Herbert V. Guenther and Leslie S. Kawamura, Dharma Publishing, Emeryville, California, 1975

Herman, Judith, *Trauma & Recovery*, Harper Collins, New York, 1997

Heyn, Birgit, *Ayurvedic Medicine: The Gentle Strength of Indian Healing*, Thorsons Publishing Group, Rochester, Vermont, 1987

The books of Johari, Harish, including *The Healing Cuisine: India's Art of Ayurvedic Cooking*, Healing Arts Press, Rochester, Vermont, 1994. Many fine works from this author.

Jones, Marjorie Hurt, *The Allergy Self-Help Cookbook*, Rodale Press, Emmaus, PA, 1984

Joshi, Sunil V., *Ayurveda and Panchakarma: The Science of Healing and Rejuvenation*, Lotus Press, Twin Lakes, WI, 1997

Kraftsow, Gary, *Yoga for Wellness: Healing with the Timeless Teachings of Viniyoga*, Penguin/Arkana, New York, 1999

Kushi, Michio, with Alex Jack, *The Cancer Prevention Diet*, St. Martin's Press, New York, 1983

Lad, Usha and Vasant, *Ayurvedic Cooking for Self-Healing*, The Ayurvedic Press, Albuquerque, NM, 1994

Lad, Vasant D., *Ayurveda: The Science of Self-Healing*, Lotus Press, Twin Lakes, 1984

Lad, Vasant D., *The Complete Book of Ayurvedic Home Remedies*, Harmony Books, New York, 1998

Lad, Vasant, and David Frawley, *The Yoga of Herbs: An Ayurvedic Guide to Herbal Medicine*, Lotus Press, Twin Lakes, WI, 1986

Lee, Charmaine, Gong of Four (Charmaine Lee, Roger Piantadosi, et al), *SynergyDance* audio and videotape, Grace Notes, 7014 Braeburn Place, Bethesda, MD 20817, (202) 363-4664

Lele, Avinash, and Subhash Ranade and David Frawley, *Secrets of Marma: A comprehensive text book of Ayurvedic vital points*, International Academy of Ayurveda, Atrey Rugnalaya, Erandawana, Pune - 411004, India, 1999

Lerner, Michael, *Choices in Healing: Integrating the Best of Conventional and Complementary Approaches to Cancer*, The MIT Press, Cambridge, MA, 1994

Levine, Peter A. with Ann Frederick, *Waking the Tiger: Healing Trauma*, North Atlantic Books, Berkeley, CA, 1997. If you start with section IV first, First Aid for Trauma, this could be one easier way to begin to grasp this valuable body-centered therapy.

Lipton, Eleanora and Alexandra Faer Bryan, *The Therapeutic Art of Polarity: An Instructional Manual for the Associate Polarity Practitioner*, Atlanta Polarity Center, 566 Pharr Road, Atlanta. GA, 30305

Madison, Deborah, *Vegetarian Cooking for Everyone*, Broadway Books, NY, NY, 1997

Morningstar, Amadea, *Ayurvedic Cooking for Westerners*, Lotus Press, Twin Lakes, WI, 1995

Morningstar, Amadea and Urmila Desai, *The Ayurvedic Cookbook*, Lotus Press, Twin Lakes, WI, 1990

Morrison, Judith, *The Book of Ayurveda: A Holistic Approach to Health and Longevity*, Simon & Schuster, New York, 1995

The Murrieta Foundation, *Murrieta Hot Springs Vegetarian Cookbook*, The Book Publishing Company, Summertown, Tennessee, 1987

Nadkarni, K.M., *Indian Materia Medica*, Popular Prakashan, Bombay, India, 1976

Packard, Candis Cantin, *Pocket Guide to Ayurvedic Healing*, The Crossing Press, Freedom, California, 1996

Perera, Sylvia Brinton, *Descent to the Goddess: A Way of Initiation for Women*, Inner City Books, Toronto, CANADA, 1981

Perera, Sylvia Brinton, *Queen Maeve and Her Lovers: A Celtic Archetype of Ectasy, Addiction, and Healing*, Carrowmore Books, New York, 1999

Pert, Candace, *Molecules of Emotion*, Touchstone, New York, New York, 1997

Peterson, Gayle, *Birthing Normally: A Personal Growth Approach to Childbirth*, second ed., MindBody Press, Berkeley, CA, 1984

Pitchford, Paul, *Healing with Whole Foods*, North Atlantic Books, Berkeley, California, 1993

Potts, Phyllis, *Going Against the Grain: Wheat-Free Cookery*, Central Point Publishing, Oregon City, OR

Ranade, Subhash, *Natural Healing through Ayurveda*, Passage Press, Salt Lake City, Utah, 1993

Rapgay, Lopsang, *The Tibetan Book of Healing*, Passage Press, Salt Lake City , Utah, 1996

Rawlinson, Ian, *Yoga for the West*, CRCS Publications, 1985

Reading, Chris M. and Ross S. Meillon, *Your Family Tree Connection: How to Use Your Past to Shape Your Future Health*, Keats Publishing, Inc., New Canaan, CT, 1984

Sachs, Melanie, *Ayurvedic Beauty Care: Ageless Techniques to Invoke Natural Beauty*, Lotus Press, Twin Lakes, WI, 1994

Sachs, Robert, *Health for Life: Secrets of Tibetan Ayurveda*, Clear Light Publishers, Santa Fe, NM, 1995

Sharan, Farida, *Herbs of Grace: Becoming Independently Healthy*, Wisdome Press, Boulder, CO, 1994, integrates herbs, Polarity and iridology

Shubentsov, Yefim and Barbara Gordon, *Cure Your Cravings*, Perigee, New York, NY, 1998

Sills, Franklyn, *The Polarity Process: Energy as a Healing Art*, Element, Rockport, MA, 1989

Spignesi, Angelyn, *Starving Women: A Psychology of Anorexia Nervosa*, Spring Publications, Inc. Dallas, TX, 1983

Spiller, Jan, *Astrology for the Soul*, Bantam Books, New York, 1997

Stone, Randolph, *Polarity Therapy*, volumes one and two, CRCS Publications, PO Box 1460, Sebastopol, CA 95472, 1985

Stone, Randolph, *Health Building: The Conscious Art of Living Well*, CRCS Publications, PO Box 1460, Sebastopol, CA 95472, 1985

Sutherland, William Garner, *Teachings in the Science of Osteopathy*, Rudra Press, Portland, OR, 1990

Svoboda, Robert E. *Ayurveda: Life, Health, & Longevity*, Arkana-Penguin Books, New York, 1992

Svoboda, Robert E., *Prakriti: Your Ayurvedic Constitution*, revised enlarged second edition, Sadhana Publications, Bellingham, WA 98225, 1998

Svoboda, Robert and Arnie Lade, *Tao and Dharma: Chinese Medicine and Ayurveda*, Lotus Press, P O Box 325, Twin Lakes, WI 53181, 1995

Tarabilda, Edward, *Ayurveda Revolutionized*, Lotus Press, Twin Lakes, WI, 1997

Tarchin, *Meditative First Aid: A Doorway to Health*, Wangapeka Books, PO Box 80-141, Green Bay, Auckland 7, New Zealand, 1990

Tirtha, Swami Sada Shiva, *The Ayurveda Encyclopedia: Natural Secrets to Healing, Prevention, & Longevity*, Ayurveda Holistic Center Press, 82A Bayville Ave, Bayville, NY, 11709, 1998

Tiwari, Maya, Ayurveda: *A Life of Balance: The Complete Guide to Ayurvedic Nutrition & Body Types with Recipes*, Healing Arts Press, Rochester, VT, 1995

Tiwari, Maya, *Ayurveda: Secrets of Healing*, Lotus Press, Twin Lakes, WI, 1995

Vanhowten, Donald, *Ayurveda & Life Impressions Bodywork*, Twin Lakes, WI, 1996, of special interest to bodyworkers, works with the five energies of Vata

Verma, Vinod, *Ayurveda: A Way of Life*, Samuel Weiser, Inc, York Beach, Maine, 1995

All of the books of Susun S. Weed, including *Breast Cancer, Breast Health* (1996), *Menopausal Years: The Wise Woman Way* (1992), and *Wise Woman Herbal for the Childbearing Year* (1985), Ash Tree Publishing, Woodstock, New York

Wood, Rebecca, *The New Whole Foods Encyclopedia: A Comprehensive Resource for Healthy Eating*, Penguin/Arkana, New York, 1999

Young, Phil, *The Art of Polarity Therapy: A Practitioner's Perspective*, Prism Press, Bridport, Dorset, 1990

ABOUT THE AUTHOR:

Amadea Morningstar is learning, teaching, and writing about healing. She lives in northern New Mexico with her husband and daughter. She can be reached at:

PMB #186
7 Avenida Vista Grande
Santa Fe, NM 87505, or through her publisher.

M

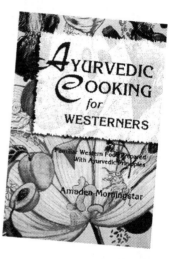

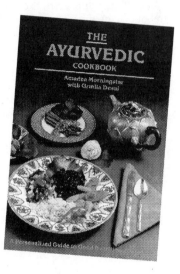

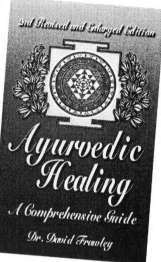

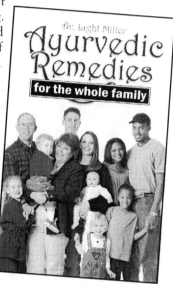

Herbs and other natural health products and information are often available at natural food stores or metaphysical bookstores. If you cannot find what you need locally, you can contact one of the following sources of supply.

Sources of Supply:

The following companies have an extensive selection of useful products and a long track-record of fulfillment. They have natural body care, aromatherapy, flower essences, crystals and tumbled stones, homeopathy, herbal products, vitamins and supplements, videos, books, audio tapes, candles, incense and bulk herbs, teas, massage tools and products and numerous alternative health items across a wide range of categories.

WHOLESALE:

Wholesale suppliers sell to stores and practitioners, not to individual consumers buying for their own personal use. Individual consumers should contact the RETAIL supplier listed below. Wholesale accounts should contact with business name, resale number or practitioner license in order to obtain a wholesale catalog and set up an account.

Lotus Light Enterprises, Inc.
P O Box 1008 AP
Silver Lake, WI 53170 USA
262 889 8501 (phone)
262 889 8591 (fax)
800 548 3824 (toll free order line)

RETAIL:

Retail suppliers provide products by mail order direct to consumers for their personal use. Stores or practitioners should contact the wholesale supplier listed above.

Internatural
33719 116th Street AP
Twin Lakes, WI 53181 USA
800 643 4221 (toll free order line)
262 889 8581 office phone
EMAIL: internatural@lotuspress.com
WEB SITE: www.internatural.com

Web site includes an extensive annotated catalog of more than 10,000 items that can be ordered "on line" for your convenience 24 hours a day, 7 days a week.